ALL INCLUSIVE DIET

ALL INCLUSIVE DIET

Finding Balance
& Keeping the
Weight Off

KRIS J. SIMPSON

NEW YORK

NASHVILLE • MELBOURNE • VANCOUVER

ALL INCLUSIVE DIET
Finding Balance & Keeping the Weight Off

© 2017 **KRIS J. SIMPSON**

Published in New York, New York, by Morgan James Publishing in partnership with Difference Press. Morgan James and The Entrepreneurial Publisher are trademarks of Morgan James, LLC. www.MorganJamesPublishing.com

The Morgan James Speakers Group can bring authors to your live event. For more information or to book an event visit The Morgan James Speakers Group at www.TheMorganJamesSpeakersGroup.com.

Neither the author nor the publisher assumes any responsibility for errors, omissions, or contrary interpretations of the subject matter herein. Any perceived slight of any individual or organization is purely unintentional.

Brand and product names are trademarks or registered trademarks of their respective owners.

The author and publisher of this book intend for this publication to provide accurate information. It is sold with the understanding that it is meant to complement, not substitute for, professional medical and psychological services.

ISBN 978-1-68350-235-7 paperback
ISBN 978-1-68350-236-4 eBook
ISBN 978-1-68350-237-1 hardcover
Library of Congress Control Number:
2016915366

Shelfie

A **free** eBook edition is available with the purchase of this print book.

CLEARLY PRINT YOUR NAME ABOVE IN UPPER CASE

Instructions to claim your free eBook edition:
1. Download the Shelfie app for Android or iOS
2. Write your name in **UPPER CASE** above
3. Use the Shelfie app to submit a photo
4. Download your eBook to any device

Cover Design by:
Heidi Miller

Interior Design by:
Bonnie Bushman
The Whole Caboodle Graphic Design

Editing:
Cynthia Kane

Author's photo courtesy of :
The Author Incubator

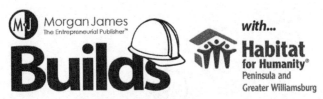

with... **Habitat for Humanity**®
Peninsula and
Greater Williamsburg

In an effort to support local communities, raise awareness and funds, Morgan James Publishing donates a percentage of all book sales for the life of each book to Habitat for Humanity Peninsula and Greater Williamsburg.

Get involved today! Visit
www.MorganJamesBuilds.com

DEDICATION

This book is dedicated to my mother who taught me life through the eyes of a librarian, George my spiritual sensei who taught me how to let go and go with the flow, Amanda who always knew this book would be born and to Josephine who proved to me that you really could keep the weight off forever.

TABLE OF CONTENTS

Introduction 1

The Story of My Struggle 10

How I Overcame Addiction and Solved My Weight-Problem 14

The 5-Facets 18

The Food Facet 24

    Food Awareness 24

    Food Journaling 28

    Math 1ˢᵗ Science 2ⁿᵈ 29

    Food Management 32

    Food Balance 42

The Emotion Facet 48

    Emotional Awareness 54

    Journaling 57

    Managing our Emotions 59

    Gratitude 61

    Social Sharing and Supporting 63

Balancing our Emotions   65

Hangriness and Tiredness   65

YOU *Time*   68

The Activity Facet   71

    Activity Awareness   73

    Arithmetic of Movement   76

    Activity Tracking   78

    Make-up Movement   80

    Activity Management   81

    Play While at Work   86

    Activity Balance   89

The Relaxing Facet   91

    Relaxing Awareness   93

    Relaxing Management   95

    Relaxing Balance   99

The Sleep Facet   102

    Sleep Awareness   105

    Sleep Management   106

    Sleep Balance   111

The Sixth Facet: Substances   114

Mistakes People Make   117

    The Top 5 Unrealistic Weight-loss Expectations   120

My Wish For You   127

Acknowledgements   131

About the Author   134

INTRODUCTION

"Why can't we keep the weight off?"

My first weight-loss client holds a very special place in my heart. I look at her as the matriarch of the weight-loss and wellness program that I now coach, *Freedom 13*. She taught me so much about why people become overweight and more importantly, how they can keep it off.

Although everyone has a unique story, there is a common thread that weaves them all together. It amazes me how similar their stories are, and it is a constant reminder that we're never alone with the unique problems we face.

Her name is Josephine, and she was 45 years old when she first asked me to help her with her weight issue. It had been a recurring problem whereby she had lost the same 50 pounds many times over since her late twenties.

I remember when I first met Josephine. She was visibly overweight, and I could tell she was trying her best to hide it through the clothes she wore. She was very friendly, but I could immediately sense that there was a lot of underlying unrest within her. It looked like she was carrying the weight of the world. I could feel the burden that Josephine was holding, and I could sense how tiresome it would be to live in her shoes.

Josephine's overweight problem was fundamentally skin deep. I could tell that she was embarrassed about her weight. This was apparent when I asked her to step on the scale. She was very reluctant and started in with a well-rehearsed script of negative self-talk. I could see that she was holding on to a lot of shame because she had gained the weight over and over again.

I got the same reaction when I asked to take Josephine's before picture. I found out that she had been avoiding pictures for years, and always dodging out of them whenever she reluctantly attended social occasions.

In fact, I found out that she normally avoided mirrors as well. She would intentionally look away or downward whenever she encountered a mirror. She even felt uncomfortable looking at herself while brushing her teeth in the morning.

Josephine wore clothes that were purposely chosen to hide the shape of her body. She told me that shopping for clothes was depressing and an embarrassing experience for her. When she was in her twenties, it was something she looked forward to, but now it was something she dreaded.

Josephine lacked confidence and self-esteem. This was sad for me because I could see that under all of that extra weight there was a beautiful woman who wasn't able to fully express herself. The extra layers of weight that she had accumulated over the years were suppressing her. Along with the extra body weight, she was also carrying emotional baggage as well.

Josephine informed me that she needed to lose 50-60 pounds. I could tell that her weight was a major concern for her, and she was serious about taking it off. I asked her why losing the weight was so important and she replied: "so when I look at my reflection in the mirror, I like what I see."

As I understood it, she wanted to regain her sense of pride and self-value. Through years of self-neglect, Josephine was finally ready to invest in herself so she could look in the mirror and feel proud and confident.

Since then I have always asked clients to tell me why losing the weight is so important to them because there's always more meaning to it than just some numbers on a scale.

In the past, Josephine would search the Internet for weight-loss programs that guaranteed results. The websites she would look at provided promising weight loss, and they all stressed the importance of diet and exercise. The quick fixes all came with strong arguments of why you would need to exclude certain foods or only eat certain foods exclusively. She bought into all of them.

I admired Josephine's perseverance to conquer this 20-year-old dilemma, but at the same time, I wondered why she kept using more or less the same methods when each time it resulted in her gaining the weight back.

I told her I felt she was in just the right mindset to finally solve this problem once and for all. When I told her this, she frowned and asked me why. I told her I believed she had reached her personal bottom where she would be willing to look at her problem from a different perspective. At this point, she would have the opportunity, to be honest, open and willing to take a new approach to the recurring issue she was dealing with.

I asked Josephine how she had tried to resolve her weight problem in the past, and it was an accumulation of mainly different diets and exercise programs. I gathered that she must have tried every diet that I had ever heard about all in the hopes of finding a solution that would take the weight off fast and finally keep it off forever.

Every diet Josephine tried seemed to work initially, but she never was able to maintain the discipline that was required to stick with it and keep the weight off. She blamed herself mainly for this and came to believe that she lacked self-discipline. She never thought that dieting perhaps wasn't the solution; in fact, she seemed fixated on her dieting beliefs, as she rhymed off all of the things she was doing wrong with her food.

Although Josephine felt better while exercising, working out didn't seem to take the weight off like she thought it would and left her feeling deflated and defeated. The exercise was considered a thing she thought she "should" be doing, but wasn't motivated to do it. She told me that during one exercise program she gained weight!

With every new diet or exercise program there was an initial success, but she always ran out of steam or something happened in her life, and it always resulted in her putting the weight back on.

Josephine also noticed that it was becoming more difficult each weight loss attempt, and she wasn't able to lose the weight as fast as she had in the past. She blamed her age for her stubborn and sluggish metabolism. She was only 45 years old, yet she was feeling rather hopeless and very frustrated.

I asked Josephine to tell me what happened the last time she lost the weight and gained it back. She told me about a crisis that had come up in her life that shook her emotionally. By the time that crisis had blown over, she was entrenched back in her old way of eating, and she couldn't get back on track.

When I asked Josephine about the times, she was successful at losing the weight, many of those programs ended because of a crisis or change that had arisen in her life, which had caused her a lot of extra stress.

Whether the life crisis was her parent was ill and in the hospital or if it were a schedule change at work, any change that caused stress in her life would knock her out of balance, and she never could get back on track. When she experienced stress, she would react by overeating, under-sleeping and not allowing herself to relax.

Josephine called herself a "stress eater" and was more than aware that her diet was dependent on her stress levels and what she was dealing with in her life. She also had a sweet tooth and constantly craved sweet carbohydrates. This is what she thought her problem was.

She gave me her deadline for taking the weight off which was three months. She would settle losing 40 pounds, but she hoped to lose 50 in 12 weeks. She had a school reunion to attend, and she wanted to fit into a certain dress. She told me she would do whatever it took to lose the weight before the event.

When she started any program, she went all in. There was always excitement and high motivation at the beginning of all the programs she tried. She always thought that this was going to be the time when she finally would solve her problem and keep the weight off permanently.

Josephine was also going through a life shift. Her children were teenagers and required less of her time. She had been working at the bank for the last 20 years. She was a manager and told me that she was very comfortable in her career, but she also told me that for the last few years she had felt like something was missing and that there was something she needed to do for herself.

She had raised two beautiful children, but she told me that it had also taken a lot out of her. She always struggled to make time for herself and was always busy trying to juggle work and family life. Her husband was busy with his career as a successful business person who was moving up the corporate ladder, and although he helped out, she was the primary caregiver for their children. She told me that although she was a proud mother, she felt as if she had missed out on a lot of her life while raising her two children and supporting her husband with his career.

Before we wrapped up our first meeting, I asked her how she would feel if she lost the weight and kept it off this time. She told me that she would feel elated, proud, happy and confident. This is what she was desperately seeking.

I then asked her what would be the first thing she would do if she lost the weight. Without hesitation, she told me she would buy the dress she wanted to wear for the school reunion.

Our journey together began after that and throughout this book I'll continue sharing her inspirational story of sustained weight loss so you can share in the same success.

Since 1995 I have been part of the fitness and weight-loss industry as a personal trainer, gym owner, and a weight-loss and wellness coach. I have helped hundreds of people just like Josephine overcome their struggle with keeping the weight off.

This book is about finding your balance and keeping the weight off. If you have taken the weight off in the past only to put it back on again, I want you to learn how to keep it off forever.

No doubt your history of taking it off and putting it back on has caused a lot of frustration, and perhaps you are very skeptical of any program that would make such a promise, but it does exist, and you might be surprised to find out what all of the other programs are missing.

You see most people think the solution is all about the science of food and exercise. It's the type of foods they eat, the time they consume them, how they combine them or the cardio they aren't doing enough of. Some of this is true, but it's only part of keeping the weight off.

If food or even combining it with exercise were the solution, then I would think that the diets you have been on in the past would have kept the weight off, but I'm assuming that didn't happen. Now it is logical to think that food and exercise are the problems and the solution, but it's not logical to continue trying different diets that never seem to keep the weight off.

We're not really to blame for this misconception because the weight-loss industry, composed of mainly diet companies, weight-loss supplement manufacturers, diet book authors and obesity doctors has been only showing us part of the truth or what's easier for us to buy into.

They focus only on taking the weight off quickly, which is an easy buy-in because it provides us with the perception of instant gratification, but it's a deception because these diets just are not sustainable.

The diets they prescribe are rigid, restrictive and unrealistic, which work initially to take the weight off quickly, but they also throw our body off balance. We take their advice, programs, and supplements in an attempt to beat our biology, but this just throws us off balance in a different direction.

Our willpower isn't enough to carry us through the strain of these unrealistic and unsustainable diets. Our cravings end up controlling us, or we feel so stifled being on a rigid diet that we want to break out and have some freedom to indulge now and then. This is the breaking point at which we then revert to the habits that caused our weight issue in the first place.

This leaves us with a tremendous amount of shame and guilt. We've failed again at having the discipline required to stick to a diet. We have failed to keep the weight off, and the worst thing is that everyone else can see that too.

This is the endless cycle that we all go through when we look at diets and exercise as the only solutions to our weight problem.

There is a bigger picture to keeping the weight off that not many people, including the entire weight-loss industry at large, acknowledge. It's time to take another approach to this problem. An unconventional approach, and after however many failures you have experienced with dieting, isn't it worth a look?

The first piece that is missing is there cannot be a difference between how you take it off and keep it off. The strategies that you are using to take it off have to be maintained. Otherwise, you won't keep it off. It makes no sense to start a diet and exercise program that you cannot see yourself sustaining in the future.

The second piece that is missing is understanding that if we can't beat our body's biology- why not work with it? If we can create balance within the body, it won't resist taking the weight off, and if the balance is maintained, our bodies will keep the weight off.

The balance that is necessary is what I refer to as our 5-Facets or F.E.A.R.S. There is a possible sixth facet for some of us that I will describe later, but there are 5-Facets that need to be balanced for us to maintain weight loss. In this book, I'll show you how to become aware of, manage and balance your F.E.A.R.S. so you can finally keep the weight off for good.

Here's a look at our F.E.A.R.S.

Food   what do you eat, how much do you eat and why do you eat it?

Emotions   do you observe your thoughts and feelings from a distance or are you reactive to them?

Activity   how do you move and how much do you move?

Relaxing   do you have down time where you participate in something that brings joy to your life?

Sleeping   are you getting enough rest and recovery?

Take the 5-Facet Lifestyle Assessment to find out if your 5-Facets are in balance, complete the 3-minute Lifestyle Assessment by visiting: www.krisjsimpson.com/lifestyle-assessment

You will find that when you start balancing all the pieces, weight loss becomes sustainable for the long-term. With this approach, you don't have to go back to another deprived way of eating and living.

Just The Facts:

A leading long-term weight loss maintenance study was conducted by The National Weight Control Registry (NWCR) They provide information about the strategies used by thousands of participants in their long-term weight loss study. According to their published report, "Research has shown that 20% of overweight individuals are successful at long-term weight loss when defined as losing at least 10% of initial body weight and maintaining the loss for at least one year." (Wing, R. Rena and Suzanne Phelan, Long-term weight loss maintenance 1'2'3'4, *The American Journal of Clinical Nutrition,* vol. 82, no. 1, pp. 222S).

I will review the top strategies that these participants used to keep the weight off throughout this book.

THE STORY OF MY STRUGGLE
"Sometimes we need a breakdown
to have a breakthrough."

W e all have wake-up calls that lead us to important life changes and transformations. If you have had any major changes in the way you live, you can probably think back to one moment when you had an epiphany whereby something happened that changed your life forever.

Some of us might have had to descend to a personal bottom before we could make the needed changes in our way of living and some of us had to hit a wall before we woke up.

My wake-up call was when I hit a wall and fell to the bottom of my front porch. It was the morning after three days of self-debauchery, which included ample amounts of what was then the substance of my former life, drugs, and alcohol.

Apparently, I had agreed to check myself into a detox center for drug and alcohol abuse. I was busily preparing myself for detox by intoxicating myself to yet another level. I regained consciousness on my front porch, and I was covered in blood. Although I was dazed and confused, I could see that I had tripped and went head first into the brick wall of my house and fallen to the bottom of the stairs.

This was what my final appearance looked like living my old life. It was the end of a 10-year progressive and painful slide into oblivion, which was written, directed and all acted out by me. The plot was a little confusing because it appeared that the main character had it all yet he was suffering.

He had so many things going for him; married with a five-year-old son and a one-year-old daughter, a successful business owner, recently moved into the posh area of town where all the big shots lived. Life on the surface didn't seem to be that bad at all.

Then why was he constantly hitting the self-destruct button?

This was the first time I honestly asked *why* and wanted to know what the answer was, no matter how painful the truth. It was the most important day of my life when I decided the show was over. There would be no more encores.

When the curtain rose again, I was locked in a detox center that I was desperately trying to escape from. I was surrounded by people who made me feel uncomfortable, but there wasn't any difference between them and me. Yes, I might have had more money and more things than most of them, but we were all under lock and key for our personal safety. We couldn't be trusted to take care of ourselves.

The week that I spent in detox was the most humiliating yet most humbling week of my life. I was at the point where my knees had hit the floor, and the only way I was going to get back on my feet again was to ask for and accept a hand.

The detox center set the stage for a one-month drug and alcohol rehabilitation program. I was open and receptive to just about any help at this point.

If I ever doubted that there wasn't a solution for the problem of addiction, all I needed to do was look around while I was in rehab and hear the stories of people who had lost it all, had risen again and had become completely transformed. Their stories inspired me and reminded me that I wasn't alone.

For a decade I had used and abused substances to create what I justified as a balance in my life. I was living life in the fast lane, across lanes, and off course completely at times.

A decade of living a life of addiction and a trail of disaster behind me, it was difficult to hide because it showed up in all areas of my life: in my relationships, my career, and it would show up later in my finances. It was also impacting my health as I was slowly deteriorating. My liver was showing the first signs of cirrhosis, and my insides were an awful mess.

What I also couldn't hide from was the fact I was 50 pounds overweight.

Fortunately, being an ex-bodybuilder I was able to justify my increase in size as muscle, but I knew otherwise. I also was able to wear athletic clothes that allowed me to hide my weight as well, but the real problem was that I wasn't real at all.

In rehab, I went through a lot of self-discovery, and I began to realize that my life was completely out of balance. I was abusing substances as a form of escape. I felt as if I needed to escape the life that I had created and which I now felt I was trapped in.

This intense state of suffering is what I call my personal bottom. I needed to go to the bottom and become completely defeated for me to hang out the white flag. My stubbornness to let go of whom I thought I was, who I thought I had to be, and what I thought I had to do showed up everywhere in my former life.

I was suffering because I felt powerless. My addiction to drugs and alcohol had taken over my life. I wasn't in control anymore. I felt like a slave, and it ate away at my soul as I lost all self-dignity and self-respect.

In rehab and more importantly in the after-care program that ensued, I got my life back to a state of equilibrium. In fact, I recreated my life to one that now serves the people I coach and me.

I share my story of struggle for anyone else who is struggling with a weight problem. It's a story about how I needed to fall to rise and live out my life legacy of inspiring others to keep the weight off and find freedom.

HOW I OVERCAME ADDICTION
AND SOLVED MY WEIGHT-PROBLEM

"Everything happens for a reason, or things
always happen then we give them a meaning. It
can mean we will become a victim or a survivor.
We have the ability to choose our destiny."

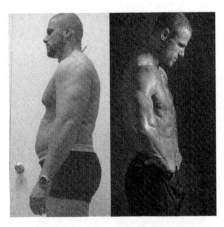

Photo Credit: Michael Fusco

Although this was very difficult for me to disclose initially, my story has become the first conversation with all of my health participants from the *Freedom 13 Weight-loss & Wellness* program, as there is a definite connection with my story and my clients' stories of struggling to keep the weight off. Through the lessons of my struggle, I can now help my clients overcome their problem of keeping the weight off.

During my recovery, I finally understood that to avoid reverting to drinking and drugging; I needed balance in my life. It wasn't so much a need as it was something that I couldn't live without. It was mandatory and non-negotiable. If I got out of balance, I knew what would happen. I would go back to drinking and drugging. It was inevitable.

I now can see the same thing happening to my clients who also have periods where their life is imbalanced, and they too are at risk of relapsing into the patterns and habits that cause them to gain weight.

I relapsed three times in the first six months out of rehab. I noticed the same pattern would occur during these episodes. Either a crisis would appear in my life that I was having difficulty managing or other things in my life would get out of whack such as working countless hours and not getting enough time to sleep and relax.

In the past when these types of things would happen in my life, I would get out of balance and turn to substances. I later learned that substances were my escape from the sense of suffering that being out of balance provoked.

My emotional imbalance had me feeling like I was on a roller coaster most days. Extreme highs followed by the bottomless lows. My exercise regimen had on and off cycles. I had no hobbies or interests to help me unwind after a long day of work. I always remember my mother asking me when I was going to find a hobby or pick up a book or start writing again. I took no time for myself, as I was dedicated to growing my business. When I did manage to find a spare moment, I was using substances to create a sense of false balance in my life. My sleep cycles were upside down because many times I didn't even know what time of day it was. This is how I now define the epitome of an imbalanced lifestyle, which was my former way of living. Although most of my clients' lifestyles are not so severely backward, they still need help with aligning their 5-Facets.

My recovery program consisted of putting my entire life back in balance one facet at a time. Little did I know that this would become the building blocks for the *Freedom 13 Weight-loss & Wellness* program.

When I started to restructure my life, I had an additional 50 pounds on my frame that I was self-conscious about. I needed to do everything in my power to bolster my self-esteem. Hence, I decided it was time to shed the baggage from my past. That baggage had to be left behind for me to move forward.

I had to look at food in a different light. I needed to take a balanced and all-inclusive approach to eating. I couldn't risk being radical, rigid and restrictive with my diet. My goal was to balance my food intake with what my body needed versus what I thought my body wanted.

Emotionally, I needed to remain balanced. I couldn't harbor grudges and hold resentments any longer. In rehab, I was taught that resentments are the number one offender when it comes to contravening sobriety. My days of arguing and complaining had to be put behind me as I needed to focus on becoming aware and managing my emotions to abstain from substances.

I had to get active again. My spirits and energy had to be sustained at the highest caliber to achieve happiness and create a new way of living. I needed to look at activity in a new and all-inclusive way. Weight training and traditional exercise were only one part of the equation, and I needed to diversify my activity so I would be more motivated to consistently engage in it.

I also needed to schedule time for relaxation. I needed to find a life outside work and find opportunities to relax, rest and recover. I never gave myself permission in the past to leave work early, but eventually, I learned how to do this without feeling tremendously guilty. I didn't find my hobbies and things to do for fun right away, but I did begin to spend more time with my children and with those I met in recovery. This allowed me to relax and reset.

Sleeping was also something that I had to take very seriously. I found that when I didn't get enough sleep, I was emotionally off balance. I felt more agitated and nervous and unable to deal with people in a calm manner. I also found that my eating got off track when I didn't get enough sleep.

Something I was taught in rehab was a concept known as *H.A.L.T.,* which stands for Hungry, Angry, Lonely and Tired. If we let ourselves get hungry, angry, lonely and tired, we run the risk of being out of balance. Hence, the term *H.A.L.T.* should encourage one to stop immediately and take a different direction or approach whenever these symptoms are experienced.

In the next chapter, I will introduce you to the 5-Facets so you can learn how to manage and balance them yourself.

THE 5-FACETS

"You will only find Freedom after you find
where your F.E.A.R.S. have been hiding."

n this section, I'm going to share with you the method I created for keeping the weight off called F.E.A.R.S (Food, Emotions, Activity, Relaxing and Sleeping). This method of addressing F.E.A.R.S. is what I use to keep myself balanced and what my client's use to keep the weight off. Before we get into each one, I'm going to share with you why these facets are so important and why they must be in balance to keep the weight off.

By definition, a symptom is any subjective evidence of disease, while a sign is any objective evidence of disease. Therefore, a symptom is a phenomenon that is experienced by the individual affected by the disease, while a sign is a phenomenon that can be detected by someone other than the individual affected by the disease.

The signs of being overweight are not the problem. The problem lies within how certain facets have become imbalanced. Our facets can be triggered by underlying issues that have not been dealt with, or perhaps we are not even aware exist. They may be in someone's blind spot, but they can still be seen as they show up in your life. We can call those symptoms.

I've discovered that being overweight is just one of the signs that there is an imbalance in life and for some of us including me that imbalance is caused by not being able to manage fear.

You can exchange the word "overweight" with "addiction" or "poor-health". All of these problems are just signs of a life that have its 5-Facets out of balance, which may or may not be caused by underlying issues that you have yet to deal with.

For some of us, it's less complicated, and it's just a matter of creating more awareness of our facets and then managing them until they are back in alignment. When this happens, the sign of being overweight disappears.

I have found through personal experience and by coaching Josephine and many other clients that no matter how out of balance one's lifestyle may have become, the managing your F.E.A.R.S. method can bring one back into balance and conclusively keep weight off.

To understand why this method works for sustained weight-loss, we only need to recognize that our body's main objective is to achieve a balanced state where all of our systems work harmoniously together. Important systems such as our metabolism, digestive and nervous systems all depend on a consistent body balance for them to operate optimally.

Because of this internal balancing system that we have within us, our bodies will constantly force us to shift back into a more balanced state because it believes its survival depends on it. Our bodies will make their corrections and at this point, you will find that if you're on a diet, it just won't work anymore.

The 5-Facets of Food, Emotions, Activity, Relaxing and Sleeping all touch each other and intersect. They all have an important role in keeping the weight off and absolutely cannot be ignored or neglected. When one of these facets is neglected, either through lack of awareness or through conscious choice, it will be out of alignment.

For example, when we don't get enough sleep, we typically overeat to compensate for the energy we don't have, or when we are in emotional turmoil, we most likely look to food to compensate for the emotional imbalance.

When one of our facets is not in balance, it creates a domino effect and throws our other facets out of balance. In this imbalanced state, it will be impossible to keep the weight off.

BEFORE WE GET STARTED!

If you haven't already completed the 5-Facet Lifestyle Assessment, I would suggest you take 3 minutes and find out which of your facets may be imbalanced so you can pay close attention to those particular upcoming chapters. To take the assessment, please go to www.krisjsimpson.com/lifestyle-assessment

Also please grab a piece of paper and a pen and answer these really important questions:

1. What goals (including your weight-loss goal) would you like to accomplish?
2. Why are these goals so important to you?
3. Have you ever tried to accomplish these goals and if yes, what worked and what didn't work?
4. How would you feel if you accomplished these goals?

At the end of each of the 5-Facet chapters, I will ask you to set a *7 Day S.M.A.R.T. SHIFT* for that particular facet. We use this approach in the *Freedom 13* program, and the results have been incredible in moving people toward their weight-loss goals.

S.M.A.R.T. SHIFT!

Introducing the *7 Day S.M.A.R.T. SHIFT,* this is an unconventional approach to goal setting and achieving consistent wins with your weight-loss. When we accumulate wins and continually achieve the goals that we set for ourselves, it keeps us in positive momentum that is critical for keeping the weight off.

Simple/Stupid - overly realistic goals

Measurable - make it super specific so you can measure your success over a seven day period

Accessible - you have everything you need to get started today

Rewardable - we typically forget to celebrate our wins and success

Team up - we need to team up for support and accountability

Simple/Stupid: It's unconventional because it takes a different approach to goal setting and achieving objectives. While many goal-setting strategies suggest that you should set stretch goals or goals that perhaps are not in your immediate reach, the *S.M.A.R.T. SHIFT* suggests keeping your goals very simplistic to the point that they almost seem to be so simple that they are "stupid" or too easy. This approach doesn't require any giant leaps and it's a goal that is well within your reach, so your probability of achieving the goal is extremely high.

S.M.A.R.T. SHIFTs also reframe your focus. Remember that we're working on a big puzzle by putting your 5-Facets back together and this will possibly be one of the most challenging lifestyle changes that you will ever work on in your life. Rather than becoming overwhelmed by these major lifestyle changes, I would like you to focus on one piece of the puzzle or one small shift at a time. When these shifts accumulate, which happens quite quickly, they progressively change the habits and patterns that are causing you weight-gain toward patterns that support keeping the weight off.

Measurable: Be sure to set some metrics and specifics to your goal so that you can measure your success over a seven day period.

Accessible: Make sure you have everything you need right away, so there is no delaying getting started.

Rewardable: Most of us never consider rewarding ourselves for the goals we achieve, but it is a very important part of the process. It can be small or big, tangible or intangible, cheap or expensive; it doesn't matter. What matters is that you reward yourself with something as it helps you identify your success and builds your confidence toward the next shift you will set. It also provides incentive, which can be a motivator that drives you toward reaching your goal. The other thing that self-rewards offer is self-care, which is something you will need to focus on because self-care is required to keep the weight off.

Team up: We are always more accountable when someone else is watching us. It's wired into our human nature. We just don't want to look bad in front of our peers so we can use this to our advantage when setting goals and team-up with someone else, a family member, friend or co-worker, and have them set an *S.M.A.R.T. SHIFT* too.

Example: My goal is to eat more vegetables on a daily basis.
Simple/Stupid—*I will eat three servings of vegetables per day for seven days.*

Measurable—*Each serving will be one cup.*

Accessible—*I will go grocery shopping today and buy the vegetables.*

Rewardable—*When I accomplish this goal I will reward myself by buying a new outfit.*

Team up—*I will ask my friend to set the same goal so we can team up.*

THE FOOD FACET

"We live with an over exaggerated abundance of
food yet we act like food is in a state of scarcity."

Why do we make food so complicated?

I would bet that you already know enough about nutrition, but what you're lacking is awareness of what, how and why you're eating. As a result, you probably do not have a suitable plan that will be a good fit for you and your lifestyle.

What you will find in this chapter is everything you will need to adapt a new way of eating that will keep the weight off with no hidden agendas. Now let's begin!

FOOD AWARENESS

When I first started coaching Josephine, she came to me and was frustrated about why she hadn't lost weight. She had started making some really important shifts in her eating and was stumped on why she hadn't lost any weight in the last few weeks. She was ready for the first exercise, which would allow her to become more aware of her food, manage, and balance it.

I asked Josephine to take a picture of her daily meals, snacks, and beverages on her smart-phone. At the end of the day, she would email me all of the pictures of her meals. I asked her to do this for one week and then we would meet again to discuss further. Although Josephine was convinced that she was eating less of the wrong foods and more of the right foods, when she started pausing before eating to take a quick picture, she became more conscious of her food and made several shifts in the one week that she was doing this exercise. When she returned to see me after one week, she was down 2 pounds. She had not lost weight in the previous three weeks so she was quite amazed by this-but I wasn't. The results are always the same; the weight magically comes off. Although Josephine believed there was something magical about it, I did not.

Most of us eat habitually. We are very much automated when we eat. Many of us are stuck in eating patterns that we've had for so many years that we're not even aware we have them. You might rush through preparing your food and eating it. You might not even have time to prepare it yourself and have to rely on take-out or highly processed foods. You might eat certain foods or just too much food because you're emotionally out of balance. While working with hundreds of health participants, I have found that they need some level of awareness before eating. Arguably, having awareness before you begin to eat would be the most important factor, and that is why Josephine had so much success with the pictorial exercise I gave her.

When I asked Josephine to take a picture of the food before she ate it, this allowed her to better prepare her meals because she knew she would have to take a picture of it and send it to me. In fact, she even went out grocery shopping to buy more suitable foods before she started this exercise! Why this simple exercise worked is because it interrupted her automated eating pattern. By asking her to stop for literally three seconds and take a photo of the food, she was about to eat it changed the way she had been doing things.

Mindful eating only requires you to develop practices that slow you down before you eat, while you eat and after you eat so you have enough time to change your choices and rewrite your automated food programming. That is what happened during the pictorial food exercise I asked Josephine to complete. She had to take a picture before she ate her food, which resulted in different food choices. She ended up breaking through the weight loss plateau she was struggling with.

It also made Josephine aware of her late night snacking habit she had been stuck in for years whereby she would graze on snack food throughout the evening. Instead of taking a serving of crackers, for example, she would take a handful, but return a short time afterward for another handful and this cycle would repeat itself a few times over the course of each night.

Taking a photo of her snack before she ate it allowed her to pull out one serving and put it in a smaller bowl instead of continuously going back for a second, third and even a fourth helping. Josephine told me that the fact she had to send me the pictures also motivated her to choose healthier evening snacks because she didn't want to look bad in my eyes by choosing extremely unhealthy food.

The simple solution would be to eat more of the right foods. However, another problem presents itself.

Are you totally aware of the food you eat? Are you aware of the following?

1. Quality
    You need to ask yourself where your food is coming from. What are their practices for growing or farming food in that country?

If you question their food handling protocols and practices, where can you find an alternative source of that food? As Oprah Winfrey said "Eating more consciously now feels like a way of being. I think about how my food got to my plate."

2. Processing

    If the food you're eating is packaged or preserved, then I would ask you to consider how it is being processed. What additional ingredients are being added? What ingredients are being removed?

3. Timing

    What time of day are you eating your food? Do you eat regularly throughout the day or inconsistently? Do you eat breakfast?

4. Combining

    How do you combine your food groups? Are you getting enough of each food group or are you deficient in some food groups and over consuming others?

5. Hunger

    Are you eating because you are physically hungry, and your body requires nourishment and fuel or are you eating out of boredom, sadness, anxiousness, loneliness or maybe because you are frustrated or angry?

6. Quantity

    Just how much food are you eating? I think you might be surprised if you were to find out.

Just The Facts:

Sited in the NWCR study "more recently, we have examined other aspects of their diet. Of particular interest is the fact that 78% of registry members report eating breakfast every day of the week. Only 4% report never eating breakfast. The typical breakfast is cereal and fruit." (Wing, R. Rena and Suzanne Phelan, Long-term weight loss maintenance 1'2'3'4, *The American Journal of Clinical Nutrition*, vol. 82, no. 1, pp. 223S)

FOOD JOURNALING

If there were only one tool or practice that I could recommend to you for keeping the weight off it would be food journaling. I have seen it make the biggest impact when it comes to keeping the weight off, yet to my surprise, so very few people practice it.

Food journaling is a practice that promotes awareness and accountability. Please note that I am not referring to "calorie counting" although that is one form of this practice. Journaling is an age-old process of self-discovery and the best tool that I know of to become aware of the what, where, when, how and why of anything we do in life.

To not be aware of what, where, when, how and why we're eating puts us in a very volatile situation where we are making decisions based on guesswork at best, or we're not thinking about it at all and running on old non-serving habits.

I have found that numerous individuals are initially resistant to investigating the facts and figures of their eating habits as they are constantly searching for the shortcut or the secret that they will discover in the next diet. This will leave them chasing the latest and greatest trends that are in an endless supply.

When you begin to food journal, you will see the truth appearing right in front of your eyes, and it brings a heightened sense of awareness. You might find that you have been eating mindlessly and without much thought and at times even when you aren't hungry. This is easy to fall into because we live fast-paced lifestyles along with an over-abundance of convenient food.

Food journaling slows you down just enough so you can reflect on what it is you are about to eat. This alone is sometimes all that is required to make the necessary changes to your diet and break the patterns that have kept you weighed down.

Journaling how you feel before and after you eat is just as important as documenting the type of food that you will be eating. You will see the connection to what degree your mood affects what and the amount of food you consume. This will give you the awareness to view yourself subjectively and be better able not to allow your feelings to dictate the food you consume.

Asking yourself where you feel your stress levels are before a meal is a practice I strongly advocate. Assign yourself a number on a scale of 1-10 of how stressed you feel and write it down beside your meal. This is also a good practice to adopt after you have finished eating as well. You can document how you are feeling physically. Are you bloated, experiencing gas or do you feel light and energized after your meal? This will give you the awareness as to what combination of foods work best for you and your digestive system. I promise you that this practice of food journaling will get you out of the dark and shed light on your issue with food, and by implementing this practice, you will already be halfway there keeping the weight off.

MATH 1ST SCIENCE 2ND

I coached a client named Genevieve who was attached to the idea that the science of the food, or the type and quality of her food, was what would keep the weight off for her. She never gave any thought to the quantity of food. She never was able to keep the weight off, though, but there was always another food trend or diet for her to believe in and the cycle of taking it off and putting it back on again. I got right to the point and asked her what the magic number was. She looked back at me very puzzled. I told her that we all have a rough estimate of how many calories we can consume per day if we want to keep the weight off.

Genevieve immediately associated what I had said with calorie counting and told me she was dead against it. I asked Genevieve why she felt that way, and she told me that when she had tried it in the past it always made her feel restricted, and it was time-consuming. I asked her to consider that she may be unaware of how many calories she is consuming. She responded, "Well not all calories are created equally." I told her I could agree with that, but if we had some awareness of the facts and figures behind her food that we would be able to manage it, and she would be able to keep the weight off. I explained this concept to Genevieve by telling her the following story:

A woman by the name of Lyn was overweight for a long time and could not seem to lose weight. She believed she was being conscious of her eating and had even started to work out two days per week to help lose weight. Lyn's weight was a big burden as it weighed her down and exhausted her. Lyn wasn't getting fulfillment out of her life because she was constantly worrying about her weight and trying to find a viable solution to losing the weight. She finally succumbed to asking for help from a professional - a Weight-loss and Wellness Coach. During their first meeting, she informed the Coach about her problem and what she had done without any positive results to rectify it. After she expanded on her story for 45 minutes, to her surprise, the Coach only had one question. "Can you provide me copies of your food and exercise logs?" The facts and figures are what the coach required more than the perception of what Lyn thought her lifestyle looked like.

After informing Genevieve of this story, she realized that there might be something in her blind spot that she needed to investigate. I set her up with one of many food logging/activity tracking apps that are available online, and she agreed to log her food. The app automatically counted the calories so she would always be aware if she were overeating within an estimated range.

What happened when Genevieve started food logging is two-pronged. First, she discovered what the magic number was and immediately knew she had been overeating based on her current activity level. And second, she became aware of the foods she was eating that contained the most calories, and she instinctively shifted toward foods that were lower in calories. What was really interesting about this exercise is that Genevieve began selecting lower calorie options, which by default were typically the healthier food choices like fruits and vegetables; in fact, her vegetable intake had tripled!

Now there has been and probably will always be opposing forces in the professional weight loss community between dietitians, fitness trainers, medical doctors and weight-loss coaches who come from different schools of thought regarding the quantity of food or the quality of food. There are some that believe that the quantity of the food we consume is not as relevant as the quality and type of foods that we eat, and there are others that believe that weight-loss is simply a mathematical and quantitative equation of moving more and eating less.

I think the truth lies somewhere between those two points of view and that's where the investigation should begin.

Just The Facts:

In the NWCR study, it stated, "Dietary intake is typically underestimated by 20–30%. Thus, registry members are probably eating closer to 1800 kcal/d. However, even with this adjustment, it is apparent that registry members maintain their weight loss by continuing to eat a low-calorie, low-fat diet." (Wing, R. Rena and Suzanne Phelan, Long-term weight loss maintenance 1'2'3'4, *The American Journal of Clinical Nutrition,* vol. 82, no. 1, pp. 223S).

FOOD MANAGEMENT

Judy was 46 when she enrolled in my program and was beginning to show symptoms of perimenopause. She was beginning to see shifts in her moods, body shape, and her menstrual cycles, which were a real wake-up call for her.

Judy told me that she had friends who barely made it through menopause because the world appeared to be turned upside down and they had a hard time coping with this natural transition that every woman goes through. Her objective was to mitigate the effects of menopause and most importantly, she didn't want to gain the 15-20 pounds which are typical for a woman going through this period of their life. I told her that I could help her by teaching her the F.E.A.R.S. method so she could be as balanced as possible before she entered the peak of perimenopause. I told her that with a specific focus on her food facet that we could create a safe passage for her.

When it comes to managing food, I always suggest that you organize it like you would anything else in your life so it becomes a personalized system that you won't have to put much thought into once menopause commences. Judy ended up losing 15 pounds after she had completed the program and most importantly, she was able to keep it off while transitioning into menopause! I would love to see other woman consider preparing for perimenopause as Judy did because way too many women suffer while they go through this life transition. Life's path is so much easier when you see what's coming and have a plan to navigate through it with ease.

Food has to move through our life, so we need to have a logistic plan so that it moves in a reasonable way. I have found a five-step logistic process to ensure that your food cycle serves you. I call it the 5-Ps to Food Logistics:

THE 5-P'S OF FOOD LOGISTICS

1. Plan—Have you sat down with a pen and paper and planned out what food you will purchase, how you will prepare it and how you will present it, so you're motivated to eat it?

2. Products—Do you use a shopping list? Do you know the simple way to read food labels and if you do, are you spending some time to look at the food labels before purchasing the food?

3. Prep—Are you prepared for your next meals in advance or are you making decisions and cooking on the fly? Do you have a simple system for your food prep that doesn't leave you desperate when it's time to eat?

4. Plate—How do you present your food? Have you ever thought that the size and shape of the food vessel would affect how much you eat? Are you using the Four Pieces of the Pie model when you are preparing your plate?

5. Palate—How does the food you prepare taste? Are you forcing yourself to eat it because you were told it's good for you and it's the only way you're going to lose weight or are you looking forward to the next meal because it lights up your taste buds?

PLAN

Failing to plan is arguably planning not to succeed. This is also true with planning our food and it's what so many of us have failed to do so it's not a surprise that we fail at keeping the weight off. We never had that plan in place to do so. This lack of a food plan and preparing to implement it leaves us at the mercy of convenient food, which in turn makes it difficult to keep the weight off. If we expect to manage our weight, we have to take back control and put together our plan that is specifically designed to meet our needs and also consider our family's needs if we don't live alone. We will need to create our food temple whereby we stock our pantry, fridge, and freezer with the food that will best serve us.

The following are some benefits of Food Planning:

✓ Save time grocery shopping, cooking, and preparing your food.
✓ Eating out less often.
✓ Less processed or unhealthy meals.

The easiest way to set up your food plan and to keep it balanced and simple is to categorize and balance your food. Although you may have been taught this model in grade school, it is the best way for the people who are interested in balancing their foods and managing their weight.

THE FOUR FOOD GROUPS:
1. Vegetables and Fruit (fresh or frozen).
2. Grain and Starches (bread, pasta, rice, quinoa, and whole-grain cereals).
3. Milk and Alternatives (milk, cheese, yogurt, kefir, soy and nut beverages).
4. Meat and Alternatives (eggs, beans, fish, poultry, lean meats, nuts and seeds).

*Fats & Sweets (there is a small allowance for foods that contain added sugar and fat in your diet).

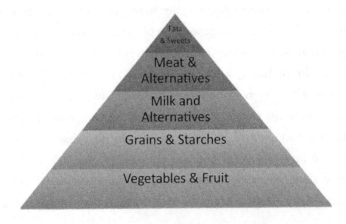

Something that is not mentioned in the food pyramid is water. How important is water? Well considering that humans are composed of approximately 60% water, it is really important to us. Another way of looking at the importance of water is to ask yourself how long you would live if you did not drink any water? On the lighter side, if we do not drink enough water, we will not be able to differentiate between hunger pangs from dehydration, not to mention experiencing lethargy. This feeling may lead to false signals that we need to eat more food to feel more energized.

I have found that most of the clients I work with are chronically dehydrated and don't even know it. They tend to drink a lot of coffee but rarely enough water. Do you know how much water you should drink per day? Well, the recommended amount of water for the average person is 2-3 liters or 60-100 ounces per day. Are you getting enough? The problem I find with dehydration is that by the time you start feeling the symptoms it's already too late. You are already dehydrated, and your body will need time to rehydrate itself. It's similar to staying out in the sun too long, by the time you feel the sunburn it is already too late. Like many of our bodily processes, losing weight requires lots of water, so if you're not drinking enough, you could be slowing down the weight loss process, and you will have an even more difficult time keeping the weight off!

Now that you have a master list of the foods you have decided you will use for your food plan you can then formulate your grocery list. This will keep you focused while you are shopping and less likely to buy food on impulse, which may not be on your master food list.

The last step is planning your meals. There is no golden rule as to some meals and snacks you should consume on a daily basis. It is completely individualized, but a general rule is that you never want to go overly hungry. If eating the traditional three square meals per day works for you then great, if you find yourself hungry between meals than snacking may be necessary for you. Remember that this is only a plan. What happens might be quite different, but that's okay because the plan is only a guide that allows you to get started. You will make many changes to the plan as you practice food awareness and understand what works for you.

*For a Free Meal Planner/Journal download, please go to www.krisjsimpson.com/free-downloads

PRODUCTS

When you have a plan, you can purchase the food products to fit your individualized plan. This is when you will need to look at your food options from the Four Food Groups, read food labels and make the most suitable food choices. You will need to educate yourself on food, but it's not as complicated as you think. Our intention is to focus on eating whole and single ingredient foods that haven't been modified by the hand of man. As my friend, Ari Whitten states in his book *Fat Loss Forever* "if it doesn't fly, swim, run or grow from the ground—don't eat it."

The fact nutrition labeling on our food products may be confusing, but if you start paying attention to the percent of daily value figures that are always included on food labels, you can make the best decisions when it's time to purchase your food. Instead of looking at the individual quantities of the nutrients, it is much easier to look at the percent of daily value to determine if food is rich in nutritional value.

THE 5-15% RULE

A general rule of thumb is that less than <5% is a little and over >15% is a lot so anything between 5-15% should be your aim for any ingredients that are important to you.

1. Start with the serving size as all the remaining facts will be based on this figure.
2. Use the % Daily value to see if the serving size has an adequate percentage of nutrients.
3. Look for the products that have more of the nutrients you want and less of the nutrients you don't want. It's as simple as that.

THE HIGH-5/ LOW-5 RULE

Another general rule is ensuring that there is no more than 5 grams of sugar in each serving and no less than 5 grams of fiber per serving.

PROCESSED PRODUCTS

The other serious and ever growing problem is the processing of our food. Now that food is in abundance for most of us in Western society it has become part of our natural expectations in life. Most of us don't give a lot of thought to what we eat. We expect it to be convenient, inexpensive, and we are not supposed to question where it originated. When we consume food that has been modified by humans or as I call it "the hand of man," we cannot expect our bodies to consume this food and continue to operate in a state of homeostasis or balance because it is digesting something that is out of balance.

Processed food is a modern day necessity, but it can also be viewed as

Nutrition Facts

Per 1 1/4 cups (58 g)

Amount	Cereal	With 1/2 cup 1% milk
Calories	210	270
	% Daily Value	
Fat 1.5 g*	2 %	5 %
Saturates 0.4 g + Trans 0 g	2 %	6 %
Polyunsaturates 0.7 g		
Omega-6 0.6 g		
Omega-3 0.1 g		
Monounsaturates 0.3 g		
Cholesterol 0 mg		
Sodium 220 mg	9 %	12 %
Potassium 210 mg	6 %	12 %
Carbohydrate 46 g	15 %	17 %
Fibre 8 g	32 %	32 %
Soluble Fibre 4 g		
Insoluble Fibre 4 g		
Sugars 5 g		
Protein 9 g		

a modern day crisis. It asks our digestive system which was wired for the food we were eating thousands of years ago to do the impossible:

1. Bypass the brain's natural food reward system.
2. Avoid overeating food that has been engineered to stimulate the reward system of the brain.
3. Digest food that doesn't resemble any natural foods.
4. Process unnatural chemical additives such as food coloring and preservatives.
5. Slow down the digestive process for food that digests quickly.

Humans have a tendency to see what they desire in something that is whole and then proceeds to single out and extract that one component. They can then form a concentrate of that one component.

Sugar is one example of this extraction and concentration process. Sugar is found naturally in beets, but can be extracted from them and refined into a concentrate that we see in common table sugar. When sugar is consumed, it stimulates the brain's reward centers because it has been exposed to something that it wouldn't find in an unrefined environment. For some individuals, this reaction stimulates the perceived need to consume more sugar.

Many processed foods have been engineered to be so incredibly "rewarding" to the brain that they overpower anything we might have come across in nature. We have complicated mechanisms in our bodies and brains that are supposed to regulate energy balance (how much we eat and how much we burn)—which, until very recently in evolutionary history, worked to keep us at a healthy weight. Reward value of foods can bypass the innate defense mechanism and make us start eating much more than we need. Processed food short-circuits our natural biology and changes our body's set point weight and body fat composition leading to the endless cycle of dieting and regaining the weight. Food manufacturers compound this problem by spending massive amounts of resources on making their foods as "rewarding" as possible to the brain, which leads to overconsumption.

THE RED FLAGS:

1. How many ingredients are on the food label? Packaged foods that have 10 or more ingredients is certainly a sign that the food has too many additives and is heavily processed.
2. Can you pronounce all of the foods on the label? If you cannot pronounce it - denounce it.
3. Beware of the Three Amigos, which are Sugar, Fat, and Salt that not only stimulate but also confuse our brains reward center.

THE GREEN FLAGS:

1. Whole grain, high fiber and low sugar food items.
2. Fresh, whole and single ingredient food items.
3. Vegetables and fruits as snack foods.

Frozen foods are sometimes a great alternative to buying fresh because although they have been preserved through freezing, they do not contain artificial preservatives that you will find in dry goods and many times they are harvested ripe since they don't have to be transported fresh. As produce is picked when it's ripe, it will contain its full nutrition potential.

*If you are considering buying organic foods, please visit this link for your free organic food report outlining the "clean fifteen" and the "dirty dozen" which will show you which fruits and vegetables specifically to buy organic, so you don't overspend on your grocery budget! **Please go to www.krisjsimpson.com/free-downloads for this free report**

PREP

Preparing your food is all about getting organized so you can implement your plan with ease. Dedicating time to prepare your food will free you up so you will not have to spend your whole day thinking or stressing about what you're going to eat next.

Here are some ideas for preparing your food:

- Freeze your food (preparing and freezing your meals will save you so much time and you will be grateful when your life gets busy, and all you need to do is simply warm up your already prepared meals).
- Prep food right out of the shopping bag (the best time to prepare your vegetables and other foods is when you arrive home from grocery shopping).
- Recipe hunting (always be experimenting and exploring with different recipes to keep your plan fresh and interesting).
- Theme nights (great for keeping it simple and consistent).
- Plan for leftovers (if you're already preparing one meal why not make enough for two or more meals while you're at it).

Where will you store the foods that you need and where will you put the foods you want? Mindful eating is about setting up cues and having the food we need visible in our kitchens. This will enable us to choose the food we need as opposed to the options we want.

PLATE

What vessel your food is placed in is something that is very subtle, but makes food logistics all that much more efficient. The plate we put our food on will determine how much food we will be consuming and allow us to divide our food into three distinct categories: meat and alternatives, grains and starches, vegetables and fruits (preferably more vegetables than fruit). This will give us the parameters for balancing our food groups and also control our consumption not eating too much food as a whole.

THE PLATE PARAMETERS

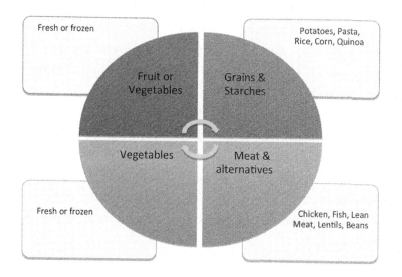

PALATE

Your food ultimately ends up in your mouth. This brings us to the final destination as far as we can see it - the palate, so it should be celebrated. Firstly, are you eating the food that you like and secondly have you put some planning and prep work into making sure it tastes good? These questions should be answered so you can have a meaningful and mindful relationship with your food.

Keep in mind that humans are always intrinsically driven to find the source of pleasurable feelings. Even our palate is set by default to find the food that makes us feel good. If you give your palate the choice, you will always be looking for foods with high amounts of sugar, salt, and fat.

The good news is that our palate can be retrained to find some pleasure in eating foods that are not high in sugar, salt, and fat, but much like training a pet, it will take some time and patience. The more vegetables and fruit we consume, the more our palate will become accustomed to the bitter and sour tastes that many fruits and vegetables have. In the opposite fashion, it will be very difficult for your palate to accept eating veggies when all it has been accustomed to is the tastes that are sweet or savory. All we need is to allocate the time and be patient with the process while integrating these foods we don't instinctively gravitate toward.

You can also create some excitement in your kitchen by experimenting and explore with different spices, new recipes, and different cooking techniques. Honestly, it can get quite boring if your food is bland so being open-minded and taking an interest to spice up your food will allow you to avoid having your palate in a state of crisis and more importantly, will keep you committed to your new way of eating.

***To download your Free Recipe E-book please go to
www.krisjsimpson.com/free-downloads**

Now that you have seen your food through its full cycle, it's time to discuss some new principles to achieve balance in your all-inclusive eating plan and to keep the weight off.

FOOD BALANCE

We need to be cognizant that stress is just a modern label we've been using in exchange for another word, which is fear. Fear is the underlying cause for all of our stressors. Food is one of our most basic needs, so under prolonged periods of stress, underlying fear is the reason that food is consumed in quantities that far exceed our needs.

The universal 80/20 principle works for eating an All-Inclusive Diet as well. I renamed it the Purpose/Pleasure principle. It simply means that 80% of the food you eat will be for a purpose, and 20% of the food you eat will be for pleasure.

The food is eaten for the purpose or roughly 80% of your food, will be clean and wholesome food that perhaps doesn't make your mouth water, but does serve its purpose of sustaining a healthy lifestyle and ultimately keeping the weight off. What this means to each will differ, but generally speaking, I am referring to food that is whole, natural and unprocessed; primarily single-ingredient foods that have not been modified by humans to a great extent.

The food is eaten for pleasure, only roughly 20% of your food, will be perhaps not the most scientifically sound food, but it will light up your taste buds and the pleasure centers of your brain. Let's face it; we're human beings, so we need to find pleasure in everything we do especially if we expect to continue doing what we're doing well into the future; so giving yourself permission to eat a small amount of food for pleasure versus purpose will light up your mouth and warm your heart. With this method of eating you can use up to 20% of your food intake as a form of daily reward. You're planning and earning your pleasure foods. This will allow you to indulge in foods that are less than perfect without packing your bags for yet another guilt trip.

When I followed up with Cathy, a graduate of my *Freedom 13* program, I asked how her diet had changed in the three years since she had completed the program and she told me that it hadn't changed at all. Although she was always experimenting and exploring with different foods, in the way she combines and cooks them, the type and quantity of her food hadn't changed much. She is still eating the same way she was eating while she was taking the weight off, the only difference now is that she's 45 pounds lighter and has been keeping the weight off for three years!

Just The Facts:

Diet consistency plays a big part in keeping the weight off as noted in the NWCR long-term weight-loss study when "Interestingly, results indicated that participants who reported a consistent diet across the week were 1.5 times more likely to maintain their weight within 5 lb over the subsequent year than participants who dieted more strictly on weekdays. (Wing, R. Rena and Suzanne Phelan, Long-term weight loss maintenance 1'2'3'4, *The American Journal of Clinical Nutrition,* vol. 82, no. 1, pp. 224S).

LATE NIGHT SNACKING

The most common problem that people have with eating healthy on a consistent basis is late night snacking. You could be having the best of eating days and completely screw up after 8:00 pm with late night snacking.

Rosanna, a client who I coached used to prepare all of her meals for the day and it, was more or less the same foods each and every day, which allowed her to have nearly perfect eating up until the evening time. She would come home after a long day and not have the willpower to prepare a healthy dinner or after dinner snacks. She also didn't have many activities to distract her from mindless late night snacking as her evening ritual was normally watching television. Between being bored in the evening and exhausted from a hard day at work, often Rosanna would derail from her healthy eating most evenings. Rosanna soon found herself stuck in a weight-loss plateau. This triggered a discussion to change her evening routine to include a walk after dinner. This allowed her to break the pattern of sitting down after she cleaned up to watch television. An extra hour of sitting was only adding to the time that she was snacking, and she found that walking helped her digest her meal and reenergized her so she could avoid the temptation of overeating in the late evening.

Here are some late night snack options:

- ✓ Soups & Salads (water rich foods have you feeling fuller).
- ✓ Smoothies & Shakes (protein based foods induce a strong anti-hunger hormone but could cause sleep disturbances).
- ✓ Popcorn & High Fibre snacks (high fiber foods foster slower digestion and provide more fullness).
- ✓ Single serving snacks (controlled portioned snacks).
- ✓ Mineral Waters (the carbonation (bubbles) can give you a feeling of being full and pose no health risks).
- ✓ Flavored Tea / non-caffeinated (a great alternative to coffee in the evening time).

Jessica, a client I coached, loved chocolate but noticed that if she ate it during the daytime, she would crave it all the way to bed that evening. I told her that she should adopt a ritual of having a single serving of her favorite chocolate right before she went to bed. I can remember her thinking that advice was crazy because she thought if she ate the chocolate right before she went to bed that it would turn into fat since she wasn't burning it off. I let her know that this was one of the many food myths, and she wouldn't have to worry about gaining weight by having a single serving of chocolate before bedtime. She liked this ritual because she found that it was an end-of-day reward that she looked forward to, and since she was going to bed right after her snack, she wouldn't be left craving more chocolate!

EATING OUT ON THE FLY

Food is an important part of every culture so having an All-Inclusive approach to food will allow you to socialize with friends and family without feeling like an outcast because you're on another restrictive diet. What is required to keep you in check and balance is a plan before you leave your environment and into the unknown? If you're going to be on the road, packing snacks are essential. If you're going out for dinner or to a function, you will need to have a plan of what you're prepared to eat and not prepared to eat while you are at the event.

Michael, a client from the *Freedom 13* program, used to spend a lot of his time in the car working as a salesperson. He wouldn't prepare food before he left the house in the morning and played the game of chance when it came to his eating plan for the day. If Michael found time to eat he would visit a take-out restaurant nearby, otherwise he would skip meals and eat one giant meal as soon as he got home from work. My suggestion for Michael was to start bringing ready to eat snacks so he wouldn't skip meals or be forced to eat fast food. Vegetables that were prepared were the easiest for him and he loved sugar snap peas and baby carrots which were ready to eat and required no preparation. I also suggested he start purchasing supplemental meal replacement bars, which he was initially hesitant about. He didn't think that eating supplement bars would be something I would recommend, and he was right in thinking so. I told him that under perfect conditions, I would love for him to always eat wholesome and unprocessed foods, but I reminded him that a day in his life wouldn't always allow for that eating so using supplements, to complement his diet would be a worthwhile alternative to skipping meals.

The following are some useful tips when eating out:

- Modify the menu—Win them with your cause!
- Hold the oil and don't bother bringing the bread!
- Order your main dish from the appetizer menu!
- Don't be Selfish - Share entrées with a friend!
- Snack before you dine!

- Doggy Bag it!
- Banish Buffets!
- Keep the Sauces on the Side!

• • • • •

Now it's time for you to consider changing your personal relationship with food. Food doesn't need to be your foe; it can be your friend. It doesn't need to be overcomplicated but instead it can be quite simple. It can be something that you consume for purpose and pleasure. It's going to require you to spend some time thinking about it, figuring out what works for you and what does not. You can consider treating food just like you treat any other relationship- with focus, attention, and love.

S.M.A.R.T. SHIFT

Now it's time to create and start your 7-Day *S.M.A.R.T. SHIFT* for the Food Facet! Please get a pen and paper so you can jot down what shift you could make to improve your eating habits!

Shift examples:

- Eating more veggies
- Preparing lunches in advance
- Cooking new recipes
- Drinking more water

What is your Simple/Stupid Shift?
How will you measure your success?
Is everything you will need accessible?
How will you reward yourself?
Who will you team up with to start this shift?

THE EMOTION FACET

"Awareness is getting out of the dark, shedding light, seeking truth and removing denial. It is the way out of Fear and the way into Freedom."

I t had been a little over three months since I had started coaching Josephine and things were going extremely well. She had already lost 25 of the 50 pounds that she wanted to lose and was now at the halfway mark, she informed me that she didn't feel like she was dieting, and in fact, she loved her new lifestyle. It belts normal to her, and she imagined she could live this way permanently.

We were working on making small, but steady modifications in each of Josephine's 5-Facets and they were beginning to compound into some incredible results. She had more awareness of her food choices, and she was no longer overeating. She was including an abundance of whole foods versus processed foods and her relationship with food was a harmonizing one. Her activity levels increased significantly as she was walking regularly. She was learning to relax by taking frequent work breaks, which included leaving the office for lunch instead of staying at the office. Her sleep had improved dramatically, and she was less stressed overall.

Although things were going really well up until this point, Josephine realized there were issues in her marriage. These issues were always there, but she had turned a blind eye toward them. She chose to suppress them for many years because she wasn't able to deal with them. As much as she wanted these martial issues to disappear magically, Josephine knew she could no longer stay in the marriage. Within a few weeks, she and her husband decided it was best to go their separate ways. This was when the storm started, and it nearly destroyed Josephine emotionally.

Josephine went through waves of emotions as she went through her separation. She experienced a combination of anger, anxiety, hurt pride, envy, resentment, and depression. I recognized how her emotional imbalance affected the balance of her other facets. As I tracked her nutrition, activity, and sleep, I could see that she was over-eating, under-sleeping and had stopped exercising entirely. Her whole life seemed to be out of balance.

This chronic emotional disturbance was slowly destroying Josephine and all that she had accomplished over the last few months. She gained 10 pounds in only a month, and I believed it was only going to spiral into further mayhem if we didn't discuss ways for her to move forward during this difficult time. I decided it was best to have a meaningful conversation.

I observed how Josephine seemed to lose herself in the emotional experience of her marriage ending. I had also gone through a similar experience, so I had a lot of empathy for her. I had taken a different approach to managing and balancing my emotions during my marriage breakup and this would be a life lesson that I would be able to share with Josephine.

I expressed to Josephine that there was only one way out, and that was to get into the eye of this emotional storm. She was confused as to what I meant, but I told her that it was the only way to find shelter and protection when the emotional storm engulfs us.

I voiced to Josephine the importance of being balanced and grounded during this emotional tempest via self-care practices. I told her that this was not the time to drown herself in her emotions. It was time for her to do something for herself. As hard as I knew that would be, I explained to her that she would need to focus on herself to feel strong and stable enough to push through this emotional storm.

This methodology would require her to invest even more into herself than she did in the past. She spent all of her time and energy worrying which left her feeling undeniably exhausted. Josephine and I worked out plans for each of her 5-Facets to get her back on track. She allowed herself time to deal with the marriage breakup, but she did not allow herself to waste time dwelling on it. She was too busy taking care of herself to be drawn into the incessant worry and insecurity that comes with not knowing what the future holds.

Josephine had a lot of pent-up anger, so we designed an exercise program that allowed her to routinely relieve her frustrations through her workouts. Although she felt resentment toward her ex-husband, we shifted her focus toward gratitude practices. These practices were incorporated into her morning rituals so she would start each day on a positive note.

The centering and calming practice that worked best to balance her emotions were the 3-minute breathing exercise that she would practice three times a day and would always resort to if she got emotionally triggered at any point of the day.

Of course, there were challenging episodes that ensued as she went through an extensive and treacherous separation process and a plethora of triggers that caused emotional upheaval. When these problems arose, I encouraged her to find answers to the cause of these triggers.

During our coaching calls, I noticed that if I brought her back to present, she could find liberation from all the fear-based emotions she was suffering from. I would continuously ask Josephine to bring her attention back to herself and away from the break-up and all the fear that it created for her, if even for a few moments; she would clear her mind and experience harmony. Occasionally, I would tell her to take a five-minute walk and call me back afterward. When she would call back, it was as if I was speaking to a different person. With a simple five-minute walk, she was a lot calmer, and her mind was clear, making it easier to work through the issue at hand.

Within four months of separation, Josephine not only got back on the path to wellness but had achieved her goal of losing 50 pounds as well. In hindsight, I knew this could have gone an entirely different direction as Josephine could have gained more weight as opposed to losing it. She may have never found the courage to face life's predicaments and effectively deal with her negative emotions that she experienced during her separation. She may have ended up remaining overweight and relentlessly searching for happiness.

We are all human, and we suffer from a similar human condition. Our condition is that we possess emotions that are constantly running through us, sometimes dictating our life. For most of us, the way we act is based on the emotions we are feeling at that moment in time.

The emotions we feel are dependent upon the thoughts we are thinking. The thoughts that we are thinking are created by our belief system or essentially what we like or dislike. At times, it is perplexing, but we need to self-manage ourselves continuously to ensure our lives are in a peaceful state.

Given that our emotional facet is the most volatile and unsteady of the 5-Facets, it will also have the most impact on our ability to keep the weight off. Our emotions should not be dismissed or ignored; they are far too important to be evaded when we are losing weight and keeping it off. Foremost, we need to be conscious of our emotions.

The problem is that most of us do not have a healthy relationship with our emotions. We may be trying to conceal them or trying to push them onto someone else. Except for joy, bliss, and excitement, most of us would rather not feel the other fear-based emotions such as resentment, jealousy, anger, guilt, shame, and sadness.

At times, we may believe that our emotions were created by some external person, place or thing. The truth is that these emotions are created within us, and it is only US who make the decision to react and respond accordingly. We can try to entomb them, but they will resurface once they are triggered by a similar experience. When they emerge, they normally have even more power over us. Our emotions become such a priority, especially when keeping the weight off.

Sometimes our emotions are not in sight. They may be in our blind spots because we put them out of sight a very long time ago. These are the most disruptive emotions that create a self-sabotaging environment and persistently control any weight-loss success we achieve.

I frequently notice that when client's emotions resurface, they sabotage their weight loss programs. I was once working with a client named Helen, and this cycle became very evident in her inability to keep the weight off. For every weight loss success high she would achieve, she would slip up which resulted in a failure to keep the weight off.

There were always reasons and justifications that she would use to explain why it happened again, but I knew there was more to it. I felt that there was something deeper that was the cause of this problem.

I decided to conduct an *emotional inventory* so we could investigate and see if there were any underlying emotions that were causing her 5-Facets to become symptomatic and ultimately out of balance. After completing an *emotional inventory* on Helen, I realized that she had a lot of emotions that she chose not to deal with.

Helen's mother, whom she was very close to, had died from cancer two years earlier. After her mother had passed away, Helen felt she had to be strong for her family. She was so strong that she didn't even allow herself to cry at the funeral. She bottled up all of the grief she experienced for the sake of being brave. Helen held a lot of pride in being strong for her family and felt that if she showed her grief that it would be seen as a sign of weakness. This grief appeared in her life as the feelings of depression and despair. When she felt this way, she became lethargic and inactive. She couldn't control her hunger cravings, so she succumbed to eating more of the wrong type of foods.

As more time passed, Helen felt she couldn't speak to anyone about how she truly felt, so she hid it until the day we had a conversation about it. It was a difficult conversation for Helen to have, but she felt a tremendous relief after disclosing what she was experiencing. Helen felt relieved after she expressed herself, but she knew she would feel even better after having a conversation with her siblings.

If our emotions are left unobserved, we may feel we are at their mercy. In Helen's situation, the balance could only be achieved once emotional disturbances were dealt with. We feel disturbances when we feel out of control; this is why so many of us are chronically out of balance and why we continue to regain the weight once we spend so much time taking it off. Every time we are emotionally triggered from perhaps a disagreement with a family member, friend or co-worker, our 5-Facets will become symptomatic. If you don't strive for an emotional equilibrium, it won't be long before this imbalance negatively affects the number on the scale.

Fortunately, there are simple solutions that if continually practiced, will bring great peace and serenity into your life. It will require strength and courage that you may have never known you had.

EMOTIONAL AWARENESS

To be completely conscious of our emotions, we need to give our full attention to the present. When we are present, we observe our thoughts and feelings from a distance, without judging them in a good way or a bad way. We call this state 'awareness' and it can only take place in the present. This is not easy for anyone to do because our emotions normally bring us back to the past or into the future, but there are some emotions that keep us right here in the present. The problem is that we have thousands of thoughts that are running through our minds each and every day. All of these thoughts, make it difficult for our mind to process information and focus on what we are doing right here, right now.

Each thought will have an emotion attached to it that we could also become attached to if we don't remain in a state of awareness. While I was on a consultation call with a client named Brielle, I saw how attached she was to one of the most delicate emotions known as resentment. During our conversation, Brielle kept referring to feelings of resentment she had against her ex-husband. He was an alcoholic while she was married to him. She blamed him for her weight problem as he created a chaotic environment for her and her children. She never had time to focus on resolving her weight problem because of the instability in their household and her life as a whole.

Every other question I asked her about herself, she referred to her ex-husband and listed all the resentments she had against him. After she had done it repeatedly throughout our conversation, I stopped her mid-sentence and brought this point to her attention. She wasn't even aware that she would mention his name every other minute during our discussion. I reminded her that this consultation was about her and not her ex-husband, so she needed to refocus. After a couple more questions it happened again. I brought it to her attention that she was doing it again, but she was not aware of her repeated behavior.

I explained to Brielle that this was completely normal, and there was nothing she could do about it, other than to be aware of it. That's it. Just be aware of it. I told her that once she became aware of this, her mind would begin to realize she was doing it. Brielle's awareness would interrupt the pattern, which would sojourn the repetitive negative dialogue of past events in her life and the resentment she harbored against her husband.

This would ultimately free up headspace, which would allow Brielle to focus on herself instead of the repetitive stories she was retelling about her ex-husband. All of that dialogue, whether it was vocalized or internalized, was distracting her from living in the moment and being present. She had to let go of the past if she wanted to focus on a future where she was a lighter and happier version of herself. There was no other way around it. Our emotions will normally anchor us in a state of the past, present or future. Emotions such as grief, frustration, disappointment, embarrassment, shame and remorse are emotions that are focused on past events and experiences. Emotions such as panic, anxiety, nervousness, envy and jealousy are emotions normally focused on the future. Essentially, it comes down to the feelings that we have for what we did or didn't do in the past or the feelings of what our imagination thinks we will be doing or not doing in the future. We can categorize all of these emotions as originating from a place of fear. They are emotions we all feel, but they are also the most dangerous emotions when it comes to making a lifelong change in body weight, these emotions have the ability to completely destroy any progress you have made with weight-loss and bring you right back to the beginning - if you grant them permission to do so.

The emotions that will stabilize and balance our minds, bodies, and the 5-Facets are focused on the present. Emotions such as joy, happiness, empathy, generosity, and gratitude allow us to focus on our well-being. They put us into a state that makes it easier to invest in ourselves, and when we begin to invest in ourselves, we begin to tackle the weight problem.

When we feel overwhelmed, it is normal because of the quantity of decisions we feel responsible for in our life. For example, saying "yes" to too many people or taking on too many things. When we become emotionally overwhelmed, I have discovered that what relieves us from our suffering is to ask ourselves, "why?" That's it. Once we do this, our minds begin to focus on the question we have asked, and it will work on it until we have the answer we have been longing for.

Everyone has what I call the anti-self or the negative inner voice that lies within us. Some of my clients vocalize their negative comments directed against themselves, and I find that when they begin to communicate these words, they have an even more damaging effect on their self-esteem. While I was coaching a small group of clients, I observed Kaya talking negatively about herself almost every opportunity she had to speak. Each time that I pointed out one of her successes, she immediately countered my compliment with a critical remark about herself. After this happened a few times, I simply asked her why was she was so critical about herself and why she wouldn't accept compliments from others. This shocked Kaya because she wasn't expecting me to ask her this question, but the second I did she began to ask herself the question and this immediately stopped her critical thinking pattern. I knew if even for a moment if I could interrupt the pattern of her negative self-talk, which she would have the opportunity to question as to why she was so hard on herself. This was a wake-up call for Kaya, and she began to call herself out whenever she had feelings of doubt that came out as either sarcastic or self-demeaning.

When we ask ourselves "why," quite often we don't have the answer right away, but in most cases, we will find it in time. The point of this exercise is to interrupt the negative emotion pattern that has been ingrained into your brain through hundreds if not thousands of repeats. The groove is so deep it's no wonder our brains fall into these patterns of thinking. It is the path of least resistance, but when you put an obstacle in the grove, your brain has no choice but to run another course. Similar to water, it always seems to find a new path.

Sometimes it might be obvious if your partner has just told you that they do not love you anymore and they are leaving you there won't be any questioning as to "why" you feel a tidal wave of emotions as you did not anticipate for them to end the relationship. There are other times that it is not as obvious, for example, when you feel anger and resentment toward your partner, but on the surface level, they have not done anything to provoke such feelings within you. So why do you feel a certain way? Why do you feel nervous? Why do you feel frustrated? Why do you feel guilty? Why do you feel powerless? Try asking yourself "why" you are feeling a certain emotion when you first feel it come on and practice being honest, open and willing while you're answering it. The trick is to catch the feeling when it first pops up in your head otherwise you might not be able to capture and contain it in the future.

Sometimes we may be unaware of the underlying emotions, but they may show up in our 5-Facets so we would want to ask: Why am I not able to sleep? Why am I so hungry and can't stop eating? Why don't I have any interest in working out?

JOURNALING

Awareness of our emotions will dictate the choices we make. It will determine how we act and behave. In my opinion, the greatest tool to bring us to the present so we can better understand our emotions is through journaling. Simply writing down how we feel.

When we take a pen and position it between our fingers, we express our thoughts and feelings on paper, which is very different from verbally communicating our thoughts and feelings. I believe this is because we can talk faster than we can write, but speed is not a feature when coming to terms with our emotions. We need space and time to explore our emotions. This process cannot be sped up, especially if you are new to self-discovery.

Setting time aside to journal in the morning or the evening is an act of discipline. Discipline begets discipline. Like a muscle, the more you exercise it, the stronger it becomes. Habits formed in one area of life have a tendency to spread; as keeping your office clean leads to keeping your bedroom tidy. Moreover, your daily practice of writing will improve other areas of your life.

After I had introduced gratitude journaling to a client named Tamera, she became focused on staying in a state of gratitude. It felt as if she had entered a whole new world, but essentially she had only changed her perception of the world through the practice of gratitude journaling. Initially, it was a tough assignment to complete, and we had to improvise to keep the flow going by adding in what could be seen as non-meaningful things like "I am grateful that the sun is shining today" but we did get a list of 10 things she was grateful for. I then asked Tamera how she felt. She paused for a moment and then said she felt better. There was some sense of relief that she was experiencing. This is not a phenomenon; it's just how our brains are programmed. If we can consider taking counter-intuitive approaches when we are feeling mad, sad or any of the other fear-based emotions, we can move into a higher state of serenity.

Before you get started with journaling, pick out a journal that is best suited for you and also decide when you will journal each day.

Here are some tips to get you started with journaling:

1. Inspiring Quotes
2. Goals you are working toward

3. Your accomplishments
4. What you're grateful for
5. Who you love

Noreen Kassam, a Psychosomatic Practitioner, has helped many of the *Freedom 13* health participants change their beliefs and thought patterns through the "W.W.I.T." or the "what would it take" journaling technique. If you are not feeling content, satisfied and happy, then how could you make a difference in the way you feel? What would it take to feel differently and if you're comfortable with how you're feeling then what would it take to continue feeling this way? You might not have answers for all of these questions initially, but that's not the point. The point is that you take the time to ask yourself these questions in the first place. As I mentioned earlier, if you are honest, open and willing to make a change, the answers will surface after you have posed the right questions. If you can begin to trust this process, even if you "fake it until you make it," you will experience profound emotional awareness.

MANAGING OUR EMOTIONS

BREATHING

Being alive is being able to breathe. Breathing is the most vital part of living because we would perish within minutes without having the gift of breath. It is this reason alone that focusing on your breath can provide you with instant gratification for relieving the daily emotional disturbances that we encounter. There is no better sense of security and safety than being able to breathe. This is why breathing is the most simplistic and effective remedy to stay in a state of freedom versus fear. We use it to regain the stability needed to manage our emotions and in essence manage our weight.

Automated within us, we normally take our breath for granted. When you are breathing shallow, this could be an indication that you are not managing your emotions and could be imbalanced. Ever since I "woke up," I have noticed how important my breathing was to keep calm, cool and collected. This habit was developed naturally through my daily meditation practice whereby deep and focused breathing is the norm. I find myself throughout the day taking deep breaths and holding it for a moment before releasing. It is now a daily ritual that doesn't require much thought, and it serves the purpose of de-stressing me.

A client named Christine used to suffer from panic attacks. Sometimes without warning or explanation, her chest would tighten to the point where she felt like she could no longer breathe. She was using a prescription anti-anxiety drug to alleviate her anxiety. I knew that breathing exercises would help relieve her anxiety, and since she had expressed interest in yoga, I suggested that she enroll in a series of classes. In yoga, breathing is an integral part of the exercise, so it's great for people who prefer an active yet gentle way of managing stress. Furthermore, breathing can put us into a higher state of awareness because our conscious mind begins to relax and focus, allowing us to feel that there are enough space and time to unwind. It is here where we can find clarity and solutions to the most challenging situations life throw at us. It is here where we can separate from our emotions and view these situations more favorably.

Socrates, a Greek philosopher, advocated the importance of controlled breathing. Socrates student's expressed to him they wanted to possess more wisdom and then asked how they could achieve such a thing. Socrates responded by saying, "follow me down to the river." He then submerged one of his student's heads underwater and released him so he could breathe again and said, "when you want to become wise as much as you want to breathe, then you will succeed."

GRATITUDE

People who can keep the weight off are a pretty happy bunch. I noticed these people naturally smile a lot more and are more optimistic as they exude a positive demeanor. Now, why is that? This is because people who have a greater sense of gratitude are typically happier individuals. When you experience the emotions of joy, empathy, generosity and love more than anger, sorrow, frustration and fear, it's much easier to keep your focus on keeping the weight off. Life, in general, is just an easier more enjoyable experience.

When we are experiencing these negative emotions, we are less likely to invest in ourselves. We eat unhealthy foods and eat too much of them. We sit more and move less. We become weighed down by these low-level emotions. As a result, releasing the weight seems next to impossible for us.

We have a choice to be happy or unhappy. How do I know? Well, I will ask you to try something that I know is impossible. Try thinking of something or someone who makes you frustrated. Once you have that thought, try thinking of something or someone who you admire and desire. Now I need you to think of both of those things or people at the same time. Were you able to think of both thoughts at precisely the same time? I didn't think so because our minds aren't designed to do that. We can only process one thought or feel at a time. This can help us express more gratitude and be like those people who are not only happier but have managed to keep the weight off. How can you cultivate more gratitude in your life?

Upon waking up or on your way to work each morning, you can prompt yourself to think of three things you are grateful for. The answers won't come right away, but you are still focused on finding something that you are grateful for so the practice is working since you can't be thinking of what you're resentful, frustrated or angry about. It is in that brief moment that your brain has an opportunity to shift from a pattern of negative thinking and start cultivating more gratitude into your life. Taking a few minutes in the morning or at any time during the day to ask yourself what you are grateful for immediately changes your mood for the better.

When you get up in the morning and perhaps again before you go to bed, list three things that you are grateful for. As with all journaling practices, they have been shown to have a greater impact when you take the time to write out your thoughts and feelings. Gratitude journaling is something you can work into your morning and evening rituals. There are also many apps and journals that you can purchase online or in a bookstore that may make it easier to sustain this practice. All of the *Freedom 13* participants use *The Five Minute Journal,* which is a simple, fast and effective way of gratitude journaling in the morning and the evening. For more info on the *Five Minute Journal,* please go to http://www.intelligentchange.com

*To download a Free *Five Minute Journal* template please go to www.krisjsimpson.com/free-downloads

Are you grateful for any particular person in your life? Telling someone you truly care about how much they mean to you has a compounding effect because now you have brought out happiness and gratitude in someone else, which in turn, makes you feel even more grateful! You can get on the phone the next time you think of them or send a quick text message. You might want to take a more personal or creative approach and send them a short handwritten note or even a thank-you card.

Just The Facts:

The importance of emotional balance and avoiding depression as a key to long-term sustained weight loss is sited in the

NWCR study, "another predictor of successful weight loss maintenance was a lower level of dietary disinhibition, which is a measure of periodic loss of control of eating. Participants who had fewer problems with disinhibition [i.e., scores <6 on the Eating Inventory subscale were 60% more likely to maintain their weight over one year. Similar findings were found for depression, with lower levels of depression related to greater odds of success. These findings point to the importance of both emotional regulation skills and control over eating in long-term successful weight loss." (Wing, R. Rena and Suzanne Phelan, Long-term weight loss maintenance 1'2'3'4, *The American Journal of Clinical Nutrition*, vol. 82, no. 1, pp. 224S).

SOCIAL SHARING AND SUPPORTING

Emotions are designed to flow through us. They are not designed to be bottled up inside. Instead, they need to be expressed. We are afraid of feeling vulnerable, so we sometimes suppress our emotions. When this occurs, our emotions remain trapped, and they prevent us from moving beyond them. However, with a little support, we can muster up the courage and share how we feel. Communicating how we feel is part of the healing process.

A client named Carol had been suppressing the resentment she had toward her husband for years. She felt that he was very controlling. Carol stated that he would frequently criticize her weight and the way she looked. Whenever she did go on a diet and started to make changes to her eating habits, he would always be very critical and didn't show any support for the efforts she was making to lose weight. Through our discussions, I discovered that Carol felt that she had purposely gained weight in the past and would sabotage any weight loss program in spite of her husband. Her revenge was based on the ill feelings she had toward him. Carol started to understand that because she was suppressing these emotions by not sharing them with others, she was purposely keeping the weight on. It reminded me of the old Nelson Mandela quote, "resentment is like drinking poison and then hoping it will kill your enemies." When Carol shared her feelings with me about this pain that she had in her life, she gained insight and began to let go. Through the course of a year, Carol released 74 pounds that she has successfully kept off for two years.

When we hide our true feelings, we create blockages that grow into heavy burdens that we carry around with us. They weigh on us literally and figuratively. We experience the same burden when we pretend to be someone who we are not for the sake of impressing our peers. It requires a lot of courage and humility, to be honest with yourself and share your true feelings with another human being. What we normally find through humility is that people become more attracted to us. There are not many brave people that can be honest with themselves and with others, so this is a way of making others feel more comfortable and safe.

When we vocalize our emotions with another person in a responsible way, we have an opportunity to both release them and also reflect on them after they have been released, so we become more aware of why we felt a certain way in the first place. This reminds me of the first meeting I had with my sponsor while I was in recovery. The words that first came out of his mouth were, "just remember that I'm here for me just as much as I'm here for you." I have learned that sometimes the best ways to get some relief from our issues is helping someone else with their troubles, which might mean just being a good listener. Remember this the next time you are fearful of sharing your emotions with another person. You may be helping them by asking them for their support.

BALANCING OUR EMOTIONS

If balancing our food is considered 80% of the solution for keeping the weight off, then our food balance will be 80% reliant on keeping our emotions in check. Have you ever experienced an emotional crisis while you were on a weight-loss program? How did it affect you? How did this emotional crisis affect your food choices, activity, and ability to relax? Did you get a good night's sleep? Were you able to manage and balance your emotions and stick with your program or did your emotions make it next to impossible to stay committed? Lastly, how did this emotional crisis affect your weight?

In almost all of the cases of people not being able to keep the weight off that I have witnessed, their failure originated from some emotional crisis that they thought they needed to attend to instead of sticking to their weight-loss program. As Janet Jackson said "When I'm feeling down on myself or not feeling good about who I am, or maybe something happened, and I'm feeling depressed, I eat to fill that void. Afterward, I'll beat myself up about it. I regret doing it, but I'll turn around and do it again."

Typically, it is three categories of life crisis that have the ability to knock even the strongest of humans off balance: relationship conflicts, career changes, and health issues. This could also be rephrased as love, wealth, and health. What I have also witnessed is that these crises can be the catalysts for change and transformation in one's life and have led many, including Josephine, to a lifetime of keeping the weight off.

HANGRINESS AND TIREDNESS

I have found that when young children are extra grumpy, it is easy to detect the problem. Most of the time, it's one of two things or perhaps even both. They are hungry and tired. They don't need a professional and hours of couch therapy to figure it out. An adult just needs to intervene and feed the child or suggest them to take a nap.

As adults, we become distracted, and we too forget that we need to eat and sleep regularly. The outcome when this occurs has been coined as "hangriness" and tiredness. If you've experienced it before, especially if you are on the receiving end, you know it's a struggle. Unfortunately, there isn't an adult to step in and rectify the situation by feeding the other adult or putting them to bed. Failing this to be your norm, you will have to develop enough awareness to know that when your emotions are starting to feel off balance, it might be attributed to missing a meal or the need to take a nap to catch up on some sleep. When feelings of emotional imbalance occur and you start to lose your patience or feel highly agitated without an apparent reason, the first question you should ask yourself: Is it time to eat?

BLOWING OFF STEAM

Many of us have a high-level of stress in our life and even more of us don't have an outlet for it. Our emotions build up and knock us out of balance. Activity is one of the most natural outlets for us to effectively release our pent up emotions, but often we stay sedentary when we're emotionally distraught instead of moving our bodies and allowing our frustrations to be released naturally.

Eckhart Tolle describes this perfectly when he uses the analogy of two ducks. Tolle said when two ducks get into a fight; it never lasts long—they soon separate and fly off in opposite directions. Each duck will then flap its wings vigorously numerous times. The ducks release a surplus of energy that builds up within them during a fight. After they flap their wings, they fly on peacefully as if nothing had ever occurred.

While I was on a coaching call with a client named Jennifer, she told me that she was feeling anxious. This was important for her to tell me because in the past when she had these feelings she would always turn to food as a sense of relief. I started to inquire with her as to the source of her anxiety, and she said "I can't put my finger on it. There's nothing in particular that is wrong; I just don't feel happy. I feel like I need to do something, or I need to be somewhere. There's this anxiety that I just cannot shake." Jennifer's situation was one I have seen many times before, and I find that when we have these feelings of discontent, we do one of two things: we try to distract ourselves with external things such as media or we mask these feelings with substances such as food or alcohol.

I have found that most of our solutions to end emotional suffering are based on our knee-jerk reaction to fight, take flight or freeze. In this example, if Jennifer were to "work" on her feelings of tension, it would elucidate the fight response. If you're feeling tense, it would be logical to put your body under more physical tension to exhaust and expand the internal tension. What you may find is that your workout may be fueled by your internal tension. You may feel better and have some relief afterward. After the rush of hormones and feel good body chemicals dissipate, you may find yourself back to feeling anxious again. This is where our underlying emotions resurface and cause recurring troubles.

I understand that balancing our emotions is not easy. In fact, being aware of our emotions is arguably one of the most challenging tasks of one's life. We are in constant communication with our inner voice, and this dictates how to act and feel. The problem is that the inner voice is coming from what I call our "anti-self" which usually doesn't provide us with the greatest advice. When we become more cognizant of our emotions, we can then feel them, identify with them, and work with them rather than against them.

YOU TIME

We spend time and do things for others to get to know them better and cultivate a strong relationship, but how much time do you spend by yourself doing things for yourself?

For most of us, there is just not enough time left because we have given it away to everyone else. We have given it away to our families, to our children, to our careers, to our friends and normally we are left with a very small window to have some alone time. To compound the issue, when we get a spare moment we are exhausted and can't do anything meaningful with that time!

When this is what our life looks like for a long period, the stress of not receiving and only giving runs us dry. When our hypothetical well is dry, we will feel very anxious, resentful and not very pleasant to be around. To balance our emotions, we will also need to make time for ourselves. When you reach the burnout point, or you can no longer manage your emotions because you are exhausted, you will require a retreat period, which many of us are reluctant to take given the busy lifestyles we lead. We will go in depth on this subject in the Relaxing Facet chapter, but you can start reclaiming some of your time now by scheduling some YOU Time!

• • • • •

When we don't manage our emotions, we become attached to them, act on them or hide from them, and they cause a lot of inner disturbances, pain, and suffering. This shows up in the other facets and as a result, they will become symptomatic or out of balance. As we now know, when we're out of balance we will show symptoms of imbalance where we feel incredibly tired or unable to sleep, hungry or without an appetite, and anxious or agitated and unable to relax.

To manage your emotions, you need to become aware of them and begin to utilize breathing techniques, gratitude, sharing and supporting.

It is only then that you can balance your emotions and in turn balance your weight. Know this is a daily practice as you will encounter things and people that will disturb and trigger your emotions. The trick is to stay consistent with these practices on a daily basis so that when your fear based emotions surface, you are better prepared to deal with them. When my clients manage their emotional lives, they can keep the weight off. No matter what diet or what exercise program they started, all of these efforts were useless until they balanced themselves emotionally.

Angela Lauria, a good friend and the publisher of this book, has the best life story to exemplify this point. Angela has lost over 100 pounds on five separate occasions. When I asked Angela what had occurred the fifth time she replied, "it took almost ten years of daily practice with the help of a coach on a consistent basis. No quick fix. No single tool. It would take a book and then some to explain. The short answer is that I became a person who didn't need to use food to manage my emotions. I ended my marriage, changed my relationship with my family and in fact, I ended almost all of the friendships that were not serving me anymore. I also left my job to become a publisher and gave up my house which incurred a cost of $100,000." In Angela's story, you can easily spot the life crisis she was facing. It wasn't until she implemented effective daily practices and reached out to a weight-loss coach that she began to manage her emotions and change her life for the better. Angela was then able to keep the weight off and live life to the fullest.

S.M.A.R.T. SHIFT

Now it's time to create and start your 7-Day *S.M.A.R.T. SHIFT* for the Emotions Facet! Please get a pen and paper so you can jot down what shift you could make to better manage your emotions, so you don't upset your weight loss!

Shift examples:

- Journaling
- Breathing Exercises
- Spending time with friends
- Spending time alone

What is your Simple/Stupid Shift?
How will you measure your success?
Is everything you will need accessible?
How will you reward yourself?
Who will you team up with to start this shift?

THE ACTIVITY FACET

"We were made to move through life,
not to sit and watch life pass us."

Before I started coaching Josephine, she went through a period where she had given up on diets. She was looking for an alternative weight loss solution, so she decided to start an exercise program. Although she never had any interest or motivation to start exercising, she knew it would be good for her and also thought that it might be a healthier way of taking the weight off. She also believed that with an exercise program, not only could she lose the weight, but also tone and firm her body at the same time.

She was driven to give exercise a shot to help her lose the weight, so she did 2-3 workouts per week. She would use the treadmill for 30-45 minutes each visit and would always feel better after she was finished, but it took a lot of motivation to get her there each time.

Josephine soon realized that she was beginning to justify eating more food than she normally would because she thought she would be able to burn it off with her exercising.

After a month of going to the gym, she was very disappointed. She had only lost two pounds. Although she did feel better, stronger and had more energy, she wasn't prepared to accept losing only two pounds per month. She needed to lose the weight much faster.

Josephine thought that if she wanted to lose more weight through exercising, she needed to do more so she decided to hire a personal trainer who could teach her how to work-out properly and increase her weight loss results.

She hired a trainer for a month and found the workouts to be very challenging. She had two workouts per week with her trainer and would just recover from the aches and pains from the last workout when she would have to complete the next one. She noticed she was working out twice as hard as she was before and felt good about herself because she was making improvements in her strength and stamina during each workout but at the end of the month she had only lost another two pounds. Josephine then decided that it wasn't working and canceled her training and membership at the gym.

Josephine's story is a common one that I have witnessed repetitively throughout my many years in the fitness business. Josephine was expecting a payback in pounds for all of the hard work she was putting in, but soon found out that exercising wasn't giving her the expected return on her investment. This is also a personal dilemma for me and every other fitness trainer or fitness club owner. People like Josephine are coming to us to solve their weight problem, but we don't have the solution.

Arguably, if the food facet is responsible for 80% of any weight you lose then exercise can only account for the remaining 20%. Our beliefs are that hard workouts will yield much more return on our investment because we feel we're investing more than we are.

When we huff, puff, sweat, moan, and groan, believing that we are putting a lot of effort into working out we then expect to see a return for this effort of equal value. Unfortunately, this is not the case. Now this might come as a surprise to you, especially coming from someone like myself, a former competitive bodybuilder, a personal trainer and fitness club owner, but I have to tell you something that you need to know: Exercise cannot be the only solution for keeping the weight off.

What we need is to move more and these days we just don't move enough. Period.

In his book, *Move a Little, Lose a Lot*, James Levine MD who is also the inventor of the treadmill desk, defines the synchronicities in the overweight and obesity epidemic in North America with our decrease in movement.

He states that Americans are in transit or their cars an average of 30 miles per day and are 30 pounds heavier than in the 1960's and that global studies show, on average, we sit 7.7 hours a day, and some results estimate people sit up to 15 hours a day. He also points out that our food may not be the only problem when he says, "there's strong evidence that our calorie consumption has gone down or at least changed minimally during the past twenty years, as obesity rates have doubled."

Most of us just don't realize how inactive we are, and we don't know how much better we'd feel and how much easier it would be to keep off the weight when we're active.

ACTIVITY AWARENESS

LOW-POWER MODE

Becoming aware of how inactive we are is normally all it takes for people to sit less and move more. In this section, I will show you what forms of movement we need to integrate into our life to keep the weight off.

Our feet were made for walking—but that's not what we do. Our bodies were made to move yet we remain sedentary. This is a fact of our modern world, which is in conflict with our prehistory bodies. Most of us are chained to our desk and on the way there and back, we're strapped into seat belts. We're still and not moving. Now, what happens to anything if it sits still for too long? Our bodies are no different.

Sedentariness has been coined the "sitting disease" and "sitting is the new smoking" has become a coined phrase. Perhaps these claims are blown out of proportion, but I believe that they make a valid point to a very serious problem.

Why are there chairs that are more expensive than treadmills? Because we're not supposed to be sitting so, chair manufacturers have had to put a lot of money into researching what chairs can make us stay comfortable in the most unnatural environment—on our butts.

Many of my clients have knee, hip and back pain mainly because they sit too much. When I got them practicing new rituals, which I outline later in this chapter, their body pains magically disappeared. A not so obvious residual benefit is that people not in chronic pain are happier and when they're happier and their emotion facet is in balance it's easier to keep the weight off.

My friend and webmaster, Steve Andrade from Digital Dabster, refers to sitting still as similar to the low power mode on your phone. When we're sitting, we're signaling to our body and mind that it's time to rest, not to be active. It's time to conserve power and transition into "low-power mode." When we're in low power mode, all of our mind and body systems go into rest mode as well. This would include our digestive system, nervous system, circulatory system and most importantly, our metabolism.

The first signal that your body will register that it needs to wake up and prepare for activity will be if you're standing and not sitting.

The second signal that your body will register is if you're moving instead of standing still. This activates all of our mind and body physiological and psychological systems and gets us into gear to perform at our best. It also activates arguably the most important physiological system that we need to lose the weight and keep it off—our metabolism!

Many times when we're feeling tired, cranky and bloated, all we need to do is get off our butts and start moving.

A client named Marion complained to me about the fact she was always feeling bloated. She was convinced it was an allergy to gluten, and she needed to stop eating wheat products. She also told me about other digestive issues she had been experiencing for years including chronic constipation. There were some periods where she wouldn't have a bowel movement for up to 3-5 days.

My intuition told me that we needed to review her activity stats and when I compiled a quick report I discovered that Marion was a very sedentary individual. She had the typical lifestyle of a two-hour commute from work where she had a sit-down desk job. She was sitting for approximately ten hours during the daytime. During her downtime, she preferred to watch television and that accounted for another 2-3 hours of sitting so in total Marion was sitting for at least 12 hours out of the 15 hours or 80% of her daily awake time. She did exercise 2-3 times per week using the treadmill in her basement, but that only accounted for an additional 1-2 hours of weekly activity. Hardly enough activity to make up for the sitting lifestyle she had become accustomed to.

Marion saw the logic in this so we agreed she would start a S.M.A.R.T. SHIFT to increase her activity and see what effect it would have on her digestive issues. We agreed she would walk for 15 minutes two times per day. We reviewed her daily schedule and decided that we would use half of the one-hour lunch break she was given at work to complete her first 15-minute walk. Marion also had a co-worker that had been asking her to go for lunchtime walks so she would take her up on the offer which would keep her more accountable and she would also be able to socialize and have some time away from her work while walking with her friend.

After Marion had completed her seven days of walking twice per day for 15 minutes, I asked her how she was feeling internally. She told me that after the third day she started feeling less bloated. Also, her bowel movements had increased from once every three days to every other day. Her energy seemed to double in the week that she started moving more and she was much happier!

When we begin moving, all of our mind and body systems are activated or turned on, and we instantly feel better. This always amazes me that when I have been sitting at my desk and writing for hours and feeling drained and tired, although I have to force myself out of the chair to go for a walk, after I return I feel re-energized. It's paradoxical that when we expend energy, we create inner energy, but that's how our bodies and minds work. They need to be turned on and in high power mode if we want them to perform at their best.

ARITHMETIC OF MOVEMENT

The complication that we have when we're overweight is that we have a surplus of calories mainly because we consume more than we burn. This surplus of calories has nowhere to go but be stored on us as body-fat. Food is a matter that contains energy. This energy either gets burned, or it gets stored.

This is the basic law of supply and demand or calorie consumption vs. calorie burn. There are too many opinions on this subject, but most weight-loss professionals all agree that we do need a balance in our calorie consumption and calorie burn and that if we are in a constant surplus state, it's highly likely that we will develop a weight problem over time.

If we move more, we burn more calories. There is a lot of factors and theories that will determine how many calories we could potentially burn like your age, weight and gender, but if we want to keep this simple and effective, we don't need to get finite about it. We just need to create a modest deficit as opposed to a state of surplus. Now let me show you how you can become more aware of the calorie economics in your life.

Calories Burned in 30 Minutes

Female—135 lbs.—40 years of age	Calories burned
House Cleaning	100
Walking (3 mph)	135
Calisthenics	135
Ashtanga Yoga	160
Dancing or Aerobics	250
Cycling	325
Running (10 mph)	550

Male—175 lbs.—40 years of age	Calories burned
House Cleaning	130
Walking (3 mph)	175
Calisthenics	175
Ashtanga Yoga	200
Dancing or Aerobics	300
Cycling	420
Running (10 mph)	700

*all figures are approximate values

ACTIVITY TRACKING

These days it's quite easy to get the feedback we need to show us if we're too sedentary. Activity trackers in all shapes and sizes are available for us to find out if we're hitting the activity targets we should be.

It's unfortunate that we need to be reminded that we should move more as it's the most natural thing we could do with our bodies, but this is the society we live in, and it doesn't look like it's going to change anytime soon. We will continue to be more distracted and more sedentary, so we need someone or something like an activity tracking device to constantly remind us to get up and move.

I have seen what I would consider the negative in the use of activity trackers with one of my clients named Leanna who became overly obsessed with reaching her activity targets. She would go to great and sometimes unnecessary lengths to achieve her activity goals. It wasn't too long into my program that she told me she couldn't manage the stress of meeting the targets and didn't want to wear the device any longer. What was happening was that when Leanna didn't hit her activity targets she would become anxious and depressed. It was becoming very counterproductive because we were also focusing on stabilizing her emotions while she was in my program. We had a long discussion about this, and I asked her to consider looking at the activity tracker for what it is—a feedback device. That's all, nothing more. It's supposed to be a guide to show you where and when you can make improvements. I also suggested that she change the targets that were set fairly high as a default to more realistic customized targets that she could not only achieve but would also allow her to achieve the goal of losing the remaining 35 pounds.

The apps of today have done a great job with using social connections to motivate a group of people to move more through various challenges that groups of people can enter. This is the accountability factor that works so well with weight-loss and wellness programs. Typically people are very concerned about their self-image and what other people think of them. There is a lot of evidence to say that this type of behavior is not healthy, but it can motivate you to pick up the pace when it comes to these activity challenges.

Most activity tracking devices use the 10,000 step model as the target for average activity. The origins of the 10,000-steps recommendation aren't exactly scientific. Pedometers sold in Japan in the 1960s were marketed under the name "man-key," which translates to "10,000 steps meter," said Catrine Tudor-Locke, director of the Walking Behavior Laboratory at Pennington Biomedical Research Center in Baton Rouge, La. The idea resonated with people, and gained popularity with Japanese walking groups, Tudor-Locke said.

Studies conducted since then suggest that people who increased their walking to 10,000 steps daily experience health benefits. One study found that women who increased their step count to nearly 10,000 steps a day reduced their blood pressure after 24 weeks. Another study of overweight women found that walking 10,000 steps a day improved their glucose levels.

On average, 2000 steps is about a mile so walking 10,000 steps means walking about five miles. How long will it take you to walk 10,000 steps? Most of us walk briskly at about 3.5 miles per hour, which takes about 17 minutes per mile or about 85 minutes for five miles.

Case in point: Most of us are not moving enough and require further awareness. How much do we need to move? I think it's safe to say that if you can move 8,000—10,000 steps per day, there is enough evidence to suggest that not only will you be much healthier; you may have also found one of the overlooked and missing pieces to solving your weight-loss problem.

Just The Facts:

An interesting fact cited in the NWCR long-term weight loss study is "Women in the registry reported expending an average of 2545 kcal/wk in physical activity, and men report an average of 3293 kcal/wk (These levels of activity would represent ≈1 h/d of moderate-intensity activity, such as brisk walking. The most common activity is walking, reported by 76% of the participants. Approximately 20% report weightlifting, 20% report cycling, and 18% report aerobics." (Wing, R. Rena and Suzanne Phelan, Long-term weight loss maintenance 1'2'3'4, *The American Journal of Clinical Nutrition,* vol. 82, no. 1, pp. 223S).

MAKE-UP MOVEMENT

Most of us, when trying to keep the weight off understand that movement is necessary. We attempt to "make up that movement" that we don't do during the day with movement mimickers otherwise known as cardio machines. There's nothing wrong with using these machines and they have a purpose for some of us, but the body doesn't respond very well to making-up. It wants constant attention and not to be ignored throughout the day.

James Levine MD states "We have evolved to hunt and gather, sow and reap, and to spend the day burning thousands of calories through constant motion, not to run like mad on a treadmill for 20-30 minutes, burning maybe 200 calories and then sit nearly motionless for the other 15 1/2 hours of the day burning next to nil."

I exercise for 30 minutes almost every day, and I believe I always will. Exercise allows us to redefine our body shape and helps us keep a healthy body image. It connects us to our bodies in a personal and deep way as we push our bodies through thresholds and beyond. We develop a relationship with our body because when we exercise we need to have that connection otherwise, we can't perform. Our bodies talk to us, and we talk about our bodies.

One thing that I understood a long time ago and I want to share with you (so you don't have to share in Josephine's frustrations) is that exercise isn't for weight-loss. It offers so many amazing benefits, but weight loss normally isn't one of them. So let's become aware of what movement and exercise are so we can have a better understanding of how we can use them to keep the weight off.

ACTIVITY MANAGEMENT

LET'S GO FOR A WALK

Walking is the most natural movement for human beings. Since the day that we decided to jump out of the trees and go for a walk, walking has been wired into us and is what is theorized as the evolution of the homo sapiens. Your feet were made for walking-not sitting. It's what we were made to do, but we don't do as much as we should.

I see walking in a much different perspective since I developed my coaching program. If you have a set of legs that work, first of all, count your blessings, and I highly suggest if you're already not walking every day to take on this activity. It's the easiest and most natural form of activity that we have to choose from.

Outdoor walking also allows us to become one with nature. Our senses pick up on the cues from nature: the colors, the smells, and the natural sounds. Seeing the grandiosity of a 100-year-old oak tree; the imperfectness of its shape still renders it beautiful; the way it bends with the wind and always recovers its true form; the sound of the leaves that brush up against each other and make a peaceful rustling sound; the breaks in the wind and the silence that follows; this is nature. This is peaceful. There is nothing like it.

3 ESSENTIALS OF EXERCISE

I am going to make an assumption about you. First, I am going to assume that you don't want to be a bodybuilder as I once was or someone who lives and breathes for their love of exercise. You may have some aspirations of being an avid exerciser in the future, but I don't think that you want to dedicate your life to it as I have. What you want is to look and feel as good as you can without having to dedicate your entire life to this vision.

If these assumptions are correct then the next section of this book will give you only the tried and true essentials of exercise so you can maximize your time, not burn out or start dreading exercise, reduce the risk of injuring yourself and continue exercising (without dreading it) for a lifetime. You always have the option of pursuing exercise as many of my clients have, but for now, it's only optional, and if you are going to invest in exercise I want you to see the maximum amount of results with the least amount of time invested.

There are three essential exercise types that I will ask you to consider including in any exercise program you do now or in the future. I would suggest doing them daily for 15-20 minutes, which you could do in the convenience of your home or at a gym if you find it to be a more motivating environment. The exercises I will recommend do not require any equipment and they are suitable for someone who is a beginner to intermediate level of fitness. They are meant to strengthen, lengthen and tone your muscles along with increasing your flexibility, stamina, balance, and coordination. This is the fun, and challenging part of this program so let's get started!

*I have created a Free Exercise Video Series to help you get started with your exercise essentials. Please go to www.krisjsimpson.com/free-downloads

CALISTHENICS

Calisthenics refers to exercises that are done in a rhythmic, systematic way using your bodyweight for resistance. Typical calisthenics exercises include pushups, jumping jacks, squats, and lunges and focus on building strength, endurance, and flexibility.

We have been taught through the influence of the classic strong man days or the more recent bodybuilding days that we need to add resistance for the movements we do to be considered exercise, but this is not true. Our body-weight, in most cases, will be sufficient resistance and something that our body structures can support. Too many times I see people using extra weight in the form of machines, barbells, and dumbbells when it isn't necessary. Your body weight combined with good old gravity will give you more than enough resistance without overstressing your muscles and joints.

What I love about calisthenics is how natural this exercise can be. It doesn't ask you to fit into a machine that sometimes feels it's made for everyone else except you. You find the range of motion that's comfortable for you and make adjustments based on your body type and how you naturally move. Because the movements are natural but exaggerated, you also (in a safe way) get the benefit of stretching while you work out as well. We call it "dynamic stretching" and it's the opposite of what is called "passive stretching." The difference is that when you're stretching your muscles dynamically, they are in motion. When you're stretching them passively, they are not in motion, so you are holding a stretch for a few seconds.

Another component of calisthenics is the core training that is commonly included. Core exercises are often looked at as abdominal training, but it goes a lot deeper than that. When referring to the core, I would like you to think about the center of your body or the trunk. As with a tree which has to withstand many natural forces like gusts of wind, the trunk is what gives the tree its flexibility and strength to counteract these forces. As with most things of integrity in life, a strong foundation, which may not be seen, is the underlying strength for any form, or in this case, your musculature. If the foundation is strong, there will be less likelihood the structure that it rests and relies on will fail. This is why I always recommend including core training with your exercise program to help avoid injury.

Have you ever suffered a pulled back muscle from some mundane chore like taking the garbage out, bringing the groceries in or shoveling the snow? Perhaps shoveling sand for my friends in the southern U.S. Often this is because our muscles are not warmed up and ready for exertion but many more times it is because we have neglected our core. Even these simple day-to-day chores require a lot of balance, stability and muscular coordination that cannot be performed optimally with a weak core.

A fact that I want you to be aware of is that you are activating your core just by standing up. In retrospect, your core is not activated while sitting in a chair or your vehicle. The core is always required and therefore activated to certain degrees if there is any body movement or any force placed against our bodies. On a side note, you're also burning three times some calories by standing versus sitting!

Core exercises can be completed with no equipment or apparatus making it very versatile and an activity that can be done at home and makes for an excellent commercial break while you're watching television!

CARDIO

Cardiovascular training is the most common form of exercising, and it offers a lot of benefits. It allows us to burn calories, strengthen our heart, improve circulation, increase stamina and lower our stress levels.

It comes in many forms:

Recreational cardio: hiking, walking, running or swimming.
Stationary Cardio: treadmill, bike, elliptical or rowing.
Group Classes: dance classes, kickboxing or boot camps.

As you can see it is very diverse, and there is a lot of room to develop it from a beginner level all the way to athletic status. Diversification is the highest recommendation for cardio for two reasons. Firstly, it is very repetitive, and if it is done on a stationary cardio machine, it can be dreadfully boring. Second, because it is very repetitive, you will be prone to overuse and injuries, which typically affect your knees and hips.

I recommend you multitask while you are doing any stationary cardio. Talk on the phone, listen to music, watch television, read, do whatever it takes to make the time go by quicker. I recommend even more that you choose recreational cardio and group cardio classes and only do stationary cardio when necessary or convenient.

COOL DOWN

After we exercise, we need to get our bodies back into balance. We have just strained them through the act of exercising, and we need to bring them back into equilibrium. The best way to do this is through a cool-down that incorporates flexibility training. This is the missing essential in so many people's exercise routines. Most people do not include a cool down into their workout because they're always conditioned to think they need to be working harder and faster and don't consider that they also need to balance this with gentle and slow movements that are incorporated in a cool down program.

Flexibility training not only prevents injuries, but it also can provide relief from any injuries you may have. A client named Sabina suffered from chronic lower back pain and a condition called sciatica. Her pain was so significant that I couldn't even advise her to walk. Instead, we set up a 10-minute stretching program that she was to do three times a day for a month. This was the only form of activity she was capable of doing, but it also had another purpose, which was to eliminate her back pain. Before the month was even up she had already reduced the pain enough to start walking. This two-step process to get Sabina active again did just that, but it also helped her overcome the back pain that was the limiter in her life.

Benefits of incorporating a cool down component to your workout:

- Relieve muscle tension
- Prevent muscle injuries
- Aid in muscle recovery (so you won't be too sore for your next workout)

PLAY WHILE AT WORK

What is the meaning of the word *workout*? My first thought is that it contains the word *work*. When was the last time you were excited at the thought of *work*? Let's compare that to other physical activities like recreation and sports for example. When we engage in sports, the saying is that we are "playing" sports—not "working" sports. Also, the definition of "recreation" is "activity done for enjoyment when one is not working". The point I am making here is that "working" out needs to be fun too, and that there has to be some "play" included for it to be considered a long-term commitment that one can maintain.

The mere fact that it appears like work makes a fitness routine a short-term perspective destined for failure (get the reward and get out). As we know, fitness is anything but short term; if you expect to keep the rewards you sowed. If you are looking to stick to an exercise program, you will need to add more play into your workouts. You can do this by including variety and human connection—two very basic human needs. Yes, exercise is repetitive work, but when you add in variety and involve other people, it doesn't seem like work any longer. It seems more like my friend and courage coach, Billy Anderson, calls a *recess*.

I have always recommended that my clients practice a sport or a recreational activity along with a regular exercise routine. I have far more confidence in these people sticking to a fitness program than the exercise fanatics who think they need to hit the gym seven days per week.

Before starting an exercise program, many of my clients are out of shape and barely have enough confidence to step into a gym. Due to this, playing a sport or some other physically demanding recreation would be out of the question for them. They have too much fear that they wouldn't be able to perform in a sport or activity like they once had, or that they didn't have the physical confidence to consider learning a sport or activity.

For many of my clients, this attitude quickly changes when they start working out and get into better physical shape. They regain their confidence to get back into sport and recreation, or find the confidence to try something new.

THE POMODORO TECHNIQUE® FOR MOVEMENT

The Pomodoro Technique® (https://en.wikipedia.org/wiki/Pomodoro Technique is a time management method developed by Francesco Cirillo in the late 1980s. The technique uses a timer to break down work into intervals, traditionally 25 minutes in length, separated by short breaks. These intervals are named pomodoros, the plural in English of the Italian word pomodoro (tomato), after the tomato-shaped kitchen timer that Cirillo used as a university student. The method is based on the idea that frequent breaks can improve mental agility.

I started thinking that this technique might be useful for a client named Sophie who was overweight and had also been in chronic pain for years.

The pain started in Sophie's ankles, went through her knees, around her hips and would then stab her in the back. She felt this shooting pain on a day-to-day basis, and it didn't end at work, it followed her home, and she would even suffer throughout the night with this chronic pain. Although Sophie hated taking pills, she had resorted to pain medication on the days that the pain was unmanageable. I introduced her to the Pomodoro method of taking productivity breaks and asked her to use it to take body breaks instead. She would put her timer on for a 25-minute cycle with a five-minute break. Every 25 minutes she would walk around her floor saying hello to coworkers and her destination would be the water-cooler. Within a week she was already feeling less pain and within a month the pain was no longer chronic, and as long as she sat less and moved more, she was able to manage her pain. Within the first year, she had achieved her goal of losing 55 pounds, and she had taken an interest in jogging. She joined a running group and after six months she decided she would enter her first short distance marathon. What a sweet success story!

ACTIVITY BALANCE

When we're inactive and sedentary, we also struggle emotionally because we always feel tired and lethargic. This can make us feel more down and depressed which will also be detrimental to our weight loss since we're now striving to maintain an upbeat and optimistic mood. Remember the body is always striving for balance and it's not working against us, it's just trying to communicate with us what it needs to stay in balance and since it doesn't speak a language per se, it will use body language or signs that if we properly identify because we're in tune with our bodies, we will be able to prevent the imbalance from continuing and throwing us off balance completely.

We also need to remember that we have a choice to create a new environment that would be conducive for our minds and bodies, and work with our biology, rather than always trying to beat them into our way of doing things. Our bodies want to stand not sit. Our bodies want to step not stagnate. To understand this concept, go for a 10-15 minute walk then ask yourself: how do I feel now? Your body will tell you that it feels energized and invigorated. I guarantee it. Here are some ideas to increase your daily movement:

- Dance (A friend of mine and the founder of the world-class entrepreneur's group Archangel Academy, Giovanni Marsico takes regular dancing breaks during the day while he's on the computer. He accredits his movement to music as being a big part of his weight-loss success story!)
- Have walking meetings
- Have walking lunches and breaks
- Park your car on the perimeter
- Take the stairs
- See housework and yard work as part of your activity program and do more of it

- Walk and talk (I use a headset for all of my coaching calls and normally reach 2,000 steps per call, and I don't even realize it!)

• • • • •

When we become aware of how sedentary we are, we finally have a chance to use our imagination and create an extraordinarily active life. It doesn't have to be complicated; it can be quite simple to start, and if you desire, you can move on to more athletic adventures with your newly aligned and active ready body. Life is always better when you're leaner, stronger and in shape. Increasing our activity one step at a time will get our bodies to this treasure filled destination and let us stay there forever.

S.M.A.R.T. SHIFT

Now it's time to create and start your 7-Day *S.M.A.R.T. SHIFT* for the Activity Facet! Please get a pen and paper to jot down what shift you could make to increase your activity and shift you in the right direction for keeping the weight off!

Shift examples:

- Talking and walking
- Exercising
- Getting 10,000 steps per day
- Taking the stairs and not the elevator

What is your Simple/Stupid Shift?

How will you measure your success?

Is everything you will need accessible?

How will you reward yourself?

Who will you team up with to start this shift?

THE RELAXING FACET

"Today I am going to forget about the rest of the world and find rest and peace of mind for myself."

When I first started coaching Josephine, she always seemed rushed and could never relax. One thing I found out later about Josephine is that she had been taking dancing lessons up until the time she went to college. She didn't have the confidence to get back into the studio and take dance lessons because she was embarrassed about her weight and didn't think she could physically keep up. I asked Josephine what she loved about dancing. She told me that dancing relaxed her so much that she would lose herself in the energy of the music. She also told me that she was in the best shape of her life when she was dancing. She felt strong and feminine, the best she had ever felt about herself and her body.

I was set on getting Josephine to partake in dance lessons, and when she became more active and took some weight off, she was ready to get started again. It wasn't long after she started dancing again that I noticed a big change in Josephine's demeanor. She just seemed more relaxed, and I believed it had a considerable impact on her weight-loss progress. One of my most cherished moments as a coach was sitting in the audience during her first dance recital.

To rest, recover, reset and reflect are things that allow us to conserve our energy, increase our focus, and help us make wiser, logical and non-emotionally driven decisions in our life. Relaxing gives us all of these things and can be defined as "the state of being free from tension and anxiety." As an added benefit, when we're relaxed, it also makes us nicer people to be around.

When we haven't taken any time for ourselves to relax, we become agitated, angry and resentful. Have you noticed these feelings when you don't have a moment for yourself and some room to breathe? With these emotions to deal with, it puts us even more out of balance.

All of these disturbances will ultimately mean one thing. You won't be able to keep the weight off. If you are always in a tense state, you're the breaking point just another disturbance away, and your self-care and weight management plan will fall apart. We can also call this a relapse because the circumstances are very similar to what I used to experience when I went back to my old ways and fell off the bandwagon.

In this chapter, we will explore the Relaxing-Facet and how it plays a significant role in keeping the weight off.

Do you find that sometimes you are afraid to take a time-out? It's counterintuitive in our culture to think that taking a timeout may help us solve any problems that we are confronted with. We are taught to believe we need to stay in the problem and work it out, don't give up, push harder and make it work.

I remember a client of mine named Alex who was running a business and rarely took time for himself to relax. He had taken on a lot of responsibilities in his life, and the pressure was on him to constantly succeed.

I decided that I wouldn't ask him to explore traditional practices of relaxation. He didn't seem like the kind of guy that would slip on a pair of tights and take a yoga class, so I asked him when did he feel the most relaxed and more importantly, what was he doing?

Alex told me that the only time he felt relaxed was while watching his sons play hockey. Although he did his best to make it to most of their games, many times Alex chose to miss them because he had to attend meetings.

I then asked Alex why he felt relaxed while watching his sons play and he told me that when they were on the ice, everything that seemed so important in his business life wasn't as important as he believed. Alex stopped thinking, worrying and projecting about all the moving parts in his business. Alex was finally focused on one thing that was very important to him, which was being present for his children and supporting them.

When Alex made it to his son's games, he also didn't have to deal with the underlying anxiety that he would always feel when he missed one of their games. Alex knew they understood why he couldn't make it, but deep down he felt very guilty about not being there.

As Alex watched more hockey games, he was getting more restful sleep and his late night snacking was more in control. I attribute this to being one of the most important shifts for Alex on his way to losing 55 pounds in six months.

RELAXING AWARENESS

I want to ask you one of the most important questions I ask all of the clients I coach when they first get started with my program.

What have you done for yourself lately?

Typically, when we engage in relaxing activities, they tend to benefit us alone, but many of us have developed a selfish complex in our society, which means that we're afraid to do anything for ourselves in fear of appearing selfish to others. This makes it very difficult to grant ourselves permission to take a load off once in awhile.

Many of us are afraid to take a day off of work, ask our spouse or family members to look after our children while we do something for ourselves or even give ourselves five minutes of solitude in a day so we can recharge our batteries. We seem to be afraid even to turn our phones off for fear that we may miss a beat of somebody else's life or their demands for us in their lives.

Either we take the pail ourselves and start refilling our well or the well will run dry. We need to reclaim some of our time so we can have time to relax. Our weight-loss success is dependent on it.

Assuming that you have failed to keep the weight off in the past, I think you will agree with me that managing your weight is probably one of the biggest challenges in your life. Well, first of all, you're not alone. Other than perhaps some very rare and genetically gifted individuals, most of us have to focus and work on maintaining our goal weight.

It may appear that some people don't have to focus on it as much as you, but in most cases, that's only because they've already done the work that I hope you will begin to do after reading this book.

If you know anyone that has kept the weight off (because they are out there), I can tell you the reason most of them make keeping the weight off look easy is because they're relaxed. They're relaxed because they take time for themselves to do the things that are important to them.

They might not be important to everyone else including their children, spouse, and boss, but they understand if they don't take that time to relax and do something for themselves they won't be able to serve these people to their fullest ability.

When you can't serve people that matter the most to your level of expectation, you will begin to feel guilty. It's at this point that you won't look relaxed anymore, and this is also when you won't be able to keep the weight off.

RELAXING MANAGEMENT

The obstacle for most of us is that we just don't have any time to relax. This poses a real dilemma because how can you manage something that we tell ourselves we don't have time for. This is where we will need to consider putting ourselves first and for many of us there is only one time of day that this could be possible– first thing in the morning.

YOUR MORNING RITUAL

Getting in front of things and preventing a problem before it happens is ancient spiritual wisdom and also good modern day common sense. Being in front of things allows us to pre-meditate without over analyzing issues that seem to be coming up over the horizon. If we're in front of events, situations, conflicts, and crises, then we may be able to rectify them before they get to the point where we are (over) reacting to them.

How can we get in front of things? One tried and tested way is by putting ourselves first. When we put ourselves first, we are relaxed enough to manage whatever life deals us.

What do we need every day to have peace of mind? You may automatically start thinking of the external things in life that need to go our way to having a peaceful day. Consider this for a moment; perhaps we only need to get into a relaxed state of mind so we can loosen up enough to go with the flow instead of becoming tense and fighting our way upstream.

After setting up a morning plan and system with a client named Sherry, I followed up with her to see how things were different in her life and this is what she told me:

I know now that my day has to begin and end with me. I need time for myself, and I cherish every morning now! Each new day needs to start early because otherwise, I will lose that precious hour or two where I do not have any immediate responsibilities. It's so nice now that I can breathe in the morning. My children are still asleep, and my office isn't open yet so I can answer my emails later!

Would it be possible for you to stay unplugged from the external world for at least the first hour upon waking? That means not checking your email, reading the paper, surfing the net or social sites, or turning the TV on to watch the news. The minute that happens, you become sucked into the vortex of other people, things, and places.

Top Practices for Morning Rituals

1. Journal or gratitude journaling.
2. Walk, exercise or stretch.
3. Read a book or daily motivation readings.
4. Listen to audiobooks & podcasts.
5. Relax and enjoy your breakfast.

A friend of mine, Hal Elrod, wrote a best-selling booked called *The Miracle Morning* that offers some great strategies to improve morning rituals. Go to **www.miraclemorning.com** for more info.

ARE YOU IN YOUR SCHEDULE?

If you want to get something done, you need to schedule it. This becomes a problem when managing relaxing time because it's your time. We're so accustomed to giving our time away so freely to others that when it comes to booking time for ourselves, we don't have any time left. For some of us, we don't even know how to take time for ourselves or there is a layer of guilt that shows up every time we try to do so.

The objective isn't to work until we burn out, rather plan ahead and know that every day we are going to need some "me-time" to relax, recover and rejuvenate. It's not a privilege; it's a prerequisite because I'm sure you know what the consequences of burnout and dispiritedness look like.

A client named Ann had completed my program in the past, but unfortunately didn't keep the weight off. She called me up about a year after she had graduated from *Freedom 13* and let me know that she was struggling to keep the weight off and in fact, she had gained almost all of the weight back that she had lost while she was in my program.

I asked her what the breaking point was for her or what changed in her life that initiated the weight re-gain, and she told me that she had left her job to start up her own business. Ann told me that she wasn't going to give up and wanted to re-enroll in my program so she could get back on track and lose the weight she had regained.

Ann got re-started with *Freedom 13* and immediately duplicated all of the prior shifts she had made in her facets. Ann essentially started living a carbon-copy of the lifestyle she had been living before she reverted to old habits.

Ann and I both expected her to drop the weight at the same rate she had the first time. This didn't happen. In fact, her weight didn't budge much at all which was both very confusing to me and very frustrating to her.

I went through her 5-Facets and scrutinized everything she was doing or not doing. She walked and supplemented with exercise; she ate a nearly perfect whole food based diet with the odd treat here and there, and she even got at least seven hours of sleep per night. Then it appeared. Both of us had missed it because it is probably the most overlooked facet of the five. She wasn't relaxing. She was stressing. She didn't have any downtime and was getting closer to burn-out.

It took a couple of weeks for Ann to work in some time for the relaxing activities she loved to do but after the first month, she was down almost ten pounds and back on track again.

Ann's story shows how stress and emotional imbalance plays a part in the weight loss process and that to reduce our stress levels we need to give ourselves back something that we had given away. Precious time. Our time is precious because once it's gone, it's gone forever; therefore we need to take some for ourselves too.

WHAT DO YOU DO FOR F.U.N.?

The definition of a hobby is " *activity, interest, enthusiasm, or amateur pastime that is undertaken for pleasure or relaxation, typically done during one's leisure time.* "

So what activities do you have in your life today that you find pleasurable and relaxing? How much leisure time do you have in your life today?

Relaxing is about bringing fun into your life. It's not about living out your life's purpose; it's about finding pleasure in life which means it will require us to do things that are F.U.N!

Frequently: What past, present or future relaxing and pleasurable activities could you incorporate into your life on a consistent basis?

Unnecessary: What activities would you consider incorporating into your life that perhaps isn't needed but which would bring you a lot of joy?

Nurturing: What activities or hobbies would you consider to be great forms of self-care and would encourage your growth and development?

These are often the forgotten things of our youth that we used to do frequently, but lost interest in or perhaps had to give up because we didn't have time for them anymore. We considered them luxuries of our juvenescence and which we now deem to be unnecessary.

They might be passions we used to have, or they might be the passions we haven't uncovered yet. We're not only limited to our past interests because we can invent new ones. The possibilities are endless and include playing music, singing, dancing, cooking, craft hobbies, painting, writing, reading and anything else you can think of that you would Frequently do which is perhaps Unnecessary, but very Nurturing!

What makes a bad day at the office, an argument with a friend or a crisis on the horizon seem smaller and more manageable? What energizes you so you can bounce back from last night's food that perhaps you shouldn't have indulged in or the regret from yesterday's missed workout? What relaxing activities will allow you some time to reflect on these mishaps and create enough space and time to figure out how to be more effective?

Now, why is incorporating relaxing activities into your life necessary for keeping the weight off? I want you to create the life now that you will live when you've lost the weight. I want you to start living like you have already lost the weight. You see that's what the secret is and what perhaps you were missing if you weren't able to keep the weight off in the past. Remember how you take it off is how you keep it off- so why not start by having F.U.N. right now?

RELAXING BALANCE

I routinely ask people how things are going in their lives. I normally get an answer that includes the word "busy". It seems that most of us are "busy"- but busy doing what and for whom?

We all seem to be busy, but I think it's a word we use so that we don't have to step up to the plate and take responsibility. When we're busy, that means we have no choice but to continue being busy while we give ourselves permission to neglect ourselves and our weight. When we use this type of language, we sound like prisoners, like we're trapped in someone else's life and don't have any freedom of choice.

I get it, we all have responsibilities to other people, places, and things but does that mean that we take very little or no responsibility for our states of mind, body and ultimately our weight?

Time is important because they're not making any more of it- so you better take some for yourself before it's too late. When you do take it back, make that time mean something—for you and only you. This time isn't about anybody else. It isn't about what you think you should be doing. It's not about getting anywhere or becoming someone you think you should be. It's only about what you want to do. It's what brings peace, joy, and pleasure into your life.

• • • • •

When you say yes to a lot of things, you will find no time for yourself. When you do take time for yourself to relax, you may need to deal with the guilt of taking back something that was yours in the first place. This will take practice, but I promise you, it will get easier. This is also when keeping the weight off will seem like a light-hearted journey.

S.M.A.R.T. SHIFT

Now it's time to create and implement your 7-Day *S.M.A.R.T. SHIFT* for the Relaxing Facet! Please get a pen and paper to jot down what shift you would make to include more F.U.N. in your life!

Shift examples:

- Taking a bath!
- Listening or playing music!

- Coloring, Writing, Reading!
- Dancing!!

What is your Simple/Stupid Shift?
How will you measure your success?
Is everything you will need accessible?
How will you reward yourself?
Who will you team up with to start this shift?

THE SLEEP FACET

"Sleep is not a privilege—it's a priority."

Josephine chronically complained about having low energy levels throughout the day. She also suffered from constant cravings for sugary foods, especially in the late afternoons. She would eat candy and chocolate most days. We had planned for her to exercise first thing in the morning because she was too busy and distracted in the evenings. This wasn't working though because she couldn't get up early to workout. All of this was causing her to gain weight, and she was becoming frustrated and wanted to give up.

Josephine knew that the afternoon snacking on candy was going to be the biggest obstacle for her to overcome if she was to keep the weight off. She asked me if there was something she could change her diet or if there was a supplement she could take to increase her energy and lose weight quickly.

I asked about her sleep patterns, and she told me she was a night owl. She had problems getting to sleep and would normally wake up in the middle of the night and not be able to get back to sleep. She said this was her sleeping pattern since having children, and she was just dealing with it.

I also asked about her nightly evening routine. She said after finishing last minute chores; she would catch up on her emails and check the news feeds on her favorite social media sites. She also found that if she started eating candy in the afternoon that she would continue eating candy and sugary foods well into the evening and normally went to bed overfull.

I suggested that we start tracking so we could establish if she were getting enough quality sleep each night. I could quickly see a pattern of both lack of sleep and poor quality sleep. She was averaging less than six hours per night and was in a restless or awake state for one hour in some cases, which reduced her total sleep to only five hours per night on average.

Normally the solution for Josephine's weight issue would be to deprive her of the sugary foods she craved and told her to exercise more. This is how we perceive the weight problem, but as you have learned through this book, it's a bigger problem than just diet and exercise.

I knew that diet and exercise, or even recommending a fat burning supplement was not going to solve Josephine's weight problem. We needed to search for the source of the problem rather than looking at it from the surface level.

I recognized that her sleep facet was out of balance and that there was a connection to her cravings for sugary foods and her chronic tiredness. We needed to create a balance which would allow her to get the rest and recovery she required, and then her cravings for sugary foods would decrease.

The first thing we needed to look at was how she prepared for sleep. We adopted a "lights-out" intention which meant that she would do her best to be in bed by 10:30 p.m. every night and lights out by 11:00 p.m. From 10:30 p.m. – 11:00 p.m. she would read a book to prepare her for sleep.

She was used to going to bed after midnight and waking up between 3:00 a.m. – 4:00 a.m. every morning and struggling to go back to bed so this was a completely different schedule for her, but within a couple of weeks she adjusted.

The second thing we did was switch her exercise sessions to the early evening instead of in the morning. She was resistant because she was told that morning exercise burns fat. I asked her bluntly how much fat she was burning now with her morning workouts that she was constantly missing.

There was another reason that I wanted Josephine to exercise in the late afternoon or early evening. I had read studies showing that vigorous cardiovascular workouts would raise your body temperature above normal a few hours before bed allowing it to start falling just as you're getting ready for bed. This decrease in body temperature appeared to be a trigger that helps ease you into sleep.

Within one month, this two-pronged approach helped Josephine not only to take off the weight she had gained but also, for the most part, eliminated her afternoon cravings and allowed her to supplement her activity with exercising on a consistent basis.

Sleep. What most of us don't get enough of? You may have already heard that we require seven to eight hours of sleep per day but honestly, who really gets eight hours of sleep after they turn the age of majority.

How does lack of sleep inhibit your ability to take weight off and more importantly keep it off?

Here are the things you need to know if you suffer from lack of sleep and how it will affect your weight:

- Sleep deprivation has a direct link to overeating and weight gain.
- There are two hormones in your body that regulate normal feelings of hunger and fullness: Ghrelin stimulates appetite and leptin send signals to the brain when you are full.
- When you don't get the sleep you need, your ghrelin levels go up, stimulating your appetite, so you want more food than you need, and your leptin levels go down, meaning you don't feel satisfied and want to keep eating. So, the more sleep you lose, the more food your body will crave.
- When you're short on sleep, you crave sugary foods that give you a quick energy boost.
- Lack of sleep disrupts cortisol levels, the hormone which is associated with stress and belly fat. It is also associated with sleep as it rises and falls with our circadian rhythms, which control our sleep-awake cycle. When we have too much cortisol, there is a higher likelihood that we will gain weight.

With these scientific facts stacked against you, there will be no chance of keeping the weight off if you're not getting enough sleep. In this section, you will become aware of your sleep, or lack thereof, and more importantly learn how to manage and balance this facet of your life so that it doesn't interfere with you keeping the weight off.

SLEEP AWARENESS

Most of us are not even aware of how much sleep we are getting and even less know what the quality of that sleep is. Being aware of your sleep (or lack of) will allow you to find a creative solution to break patterns that are keeping you up late at night or causing your restlessness or awake periods while you sleep.

One thing that we are aware of is how tired we are. In Arianna Huffington's book "The Sleep Revolution" she points out that if you type the words "why am I" into the search field that Google's autocomplete function - based on the most common searches—finishes your thought by suggesting the phrase "why am I so tired?" She also states that "we may be what we eat, but also, to be sure, we are how we sleep."

Most activity tracking devices can track your sleep. These trackers track not only the quantity of your sleep but also the quality. They work by monitoring your motion while you're sleeping and register points during your sleep where you're restless or awake. When we're restless during sleep, we're not in a deep sleep where our bodies need to be to restore, repair, and recover.

How does late night eating affect your sleep? How do certain foods that you eat in the evening affect your sleep?

Is watching media before you go to bed disrupting your circadian rhythms? Do you have a ritual that prepares you for sleep such as reading, journaling or perhaps taking a warm bath? These are all questions that need to be answered to become aware of one of the most meaningful daily rituals that all humans must partake in- sleep.

SLEEP MANAGEMENT

DO YOU HAVE RHYTHM?

Your internal 24-hour sleep-wake cycle, otherwise known as your biological clock or circadian rhythm, is regulated by processes in the brain that respond to how long you've been awake and the changes between light and dark.

At night, your body responds to the loss of daylight by producing melatonin, a hormone that makes you sleepy. During the day, sunlight triggers the brain to inhibit melatonin production, so you feel awake and alert.

The production of melatonin can also be thrown off when you're deprived of sunlight during the day or exposed to too much artificial light at night–especially the light from electronic devices, including television, computers, tablets, and mobile phones.

To sync up with our natural biological or circadian rhythms, we need to spend more time outside during the day and less time in front of our devices in the evening time to manage our sleep efficiently. We need to start winding down when the sun sets and prepare ourselves for sleep versus winding ourselves up and not being able to fall asleep at night.

YOUR EVENING RITUAL

I have found that many people who have been successful with keeping the weight off put a lot of importance on their morning rituals. I dedicate the first hour of every morning to myself for relaxing practices and to prepare for the day ahead. We do this because we need to have enough mental bandwidth to keep our 5-Facets balanced throughout the day, and so we don't throw ourselves out of sync.

Your morning ritual is dependent on what happens the night before. Did you wind-down and relax, so you were primed to have a good night's sleep? Without a system in place or a ritual for your evenings, your morning rituals won't be effective. You might even miss them all together since you're still sleeping.

A client named Mariella would put the kids down for bed and always cherished the time she had to herself. Sometimes she lingered in it well past the time she should have gone to bed to get a good night's sleep. Being a single mother with a career didn't leave her with much time for herself, so she took advantage of it when it was most available: in the late evenings.

Most of her evenings were spent answering emails, surfing the net and spending lots of time on social media sites. She would get sucked down the rabbit hole while she was on the internet and would come out the other side sometime in the early hours of the next morning.

She didn't have much of a system to get the kids out of bed and ready for school and she was trying to get herself ready at the same time. I imagined that her mornings looked like someone had hit the red panic button and it was all hands on deck. Not the easiest way to start off the day and that was the pace and tone that was set for the rest of her work day.

At the end of the day, she was so emotionally and physically drained from running on adrenalin that she had no motivation or energy to take a walk and prepare her food for the next day. With her activity levels very low and a food plan that rarely was put into motion, she didn't lose any weight her first month in my program.

After we had known that her lack of sleep was affecting her weight-loss results, we worked on creating her evening ritual to allow her time to unwind in the evening, prepare for the next day and still get to bed on time. In the mornings she was up on time and already prepared for the next day so she would have some time to relax in the morning before she had to wind-up and start her day.

Mariella used to be an avid reader but hadn't read a book in years, but she found reading very relaxing and calming, so we set up a *S.M.A.R.T. SHIFT* for her to read in the morning and the evening with an aim to only read for 10 minutes upon waking and just before bed.

Mariella's stress levels dropped dramatically because she was getting enough sleep, had her food prepared for the next day and still had time for herself in the morning and evening to relax. This new state that she created allowed her to lose weight.

The objective for your evening rituals is simple. You need to unwind and relax and get into bed to allow yourself enough time to sleep and recover for the next day. When we don't have a system, pattern or ritual in place, we will become distracted and miss our bedtime. When this occurs, we may miss our wake-time and start our day off with the unnecessary stress that usually defines how we will feel for the remainder of the work day.

Top Practices for Evening Rituals:

1. Preparing for your next day (including your food)
2. Using the Kill-Switch method (turning off all of your electronic {distraction} devices at a certain time every night)
3. Set a time to be in bed with a buffer period to fall asleep and keep it consistent
4. Journaling (including gratitude journaling)
5. Read (on a non-digital device)

BEDTIME SNACKS

The food we eat before bedtime will affect our quality of sleep. Everyone reacts differently to eating later in the evening so it is something you will need to become aware of and self-manage. Some people cannot go to sleep on an empty stomach. This will cause restlessness perhaps to the point that they are awakened from hunger and need to have a mid-sleep snack.

One myth that needs to be addressed is that late-night snacking causes weight gain. There have been plenty of studies that show that eating later in the day does not cause weight gain, rather it would be the total quantity and quality of your food throughout the entire day that will cause weight-gain.

To avoid rehashing that argument, the relevant question you would want to ask yourself is how is your sleep affected by late night snacking? Do you feel you require something to eat before bed? If so, then what food choices are you going to make?

Here are the top strategies for getting superlative slumbers:

KEEP IT LOW-PROTEIN

You will want to avoid high protein or foods from the meat and alternatives food group for bedtime snacks. Protein is slow to digest and could cause sleep disturbances so consider eating foods from the grain and starches or milk and alternative food groups as a bedtime snack. As you can see, there is some science behind the traditional milk and cereal bedtime snack that many of us crave.

KEEP IT HIGH-TRYPTOPHAN

The type of foods that you will want to have a bedtime snack is high in tryptophan. It is a substance in certain foods that induces sleep. You may be familiar with how eating turkey induces sleep, well this is because turkey contains tryptophan, but there are other foods that contain higher quantities of tryptophan and are more suitable as a bedtime snack such as foods from the milk and alternatives food group, bananas, and honey.

KEEP IT COOL

Keep the room cool. When you fall asleep, your body temperature homeostasis or balance (temperature your brain is trying to achieve) goes down. If the room temperature is too cold or too hot, it can cause stress on the system and disrupt sleep. The typical range that works best is between 65-70 degrees F.

KEEP IT DARK

In the absence of light, the pineal gland produces melatonin, which is known as the regulator of the sleep-wake cycle in the body. It monitors sleep cycles while playing an important role in healing. Any light can interfere with normal melatonin production and negatively affect sleeping patterns. Turn off all lights, turn your alarm clock away from you and close the blinds.

KEEP THEM CLOSE

Sleeping with a partner promotes feelings of safety and security, which may lower levels of cortisol, a stress and sleep hormone and sharing a bed may also reduce cytokines, which are involved in inflammation, and boost oxytocin, the so-called love hormone that is known to ease anxiety and is produced in the same part of the brain responsible for the sleep-wake cycle.

SLEEP BALANCE

I want to point something out that's really important because your body might be sending you mixed messages about how much sleep you require. If you have become accustomed to limited sleep (anything under 7-8 hours per night), our bodies get out of their natural circadian rhythm and make adjustments for this imbalance.

If you are normally sleeping 5-6 hours on average per night, but periodically sleep for the recommended 7-8, you may feel groggy and out of balance the next day. You may then believe that getting 7-8 hours of sleep doesn't work for you. But here's a question; what if you were to get 7-8 hours of sleep for three days in a row- or maybe even a week straight? How would you feel then? If you were to shift into sleeping for the recommended 7-8 hours per night, you would then comprehend how much more balanced you feel when you're getting the suggested amount of sleep.

If you are getting the recommended 7-8 hours of sleep per night consistently, you will be more relaxed, calm and manage your stress better. Your hunger hormones will also be in balance, so you don't get into a crazed food-craving state!

When we don't get the required sleep, our hunger hormones get confused, and we tend to overeat. Most of us also have difficulty managing our emotions with the lack of sleep. You will find that you're more agitated and become frustrated more easily. You will find it challenging to be patient with people like your co-workers or your children. We also don't have that extra get up and go that we require being active. We feel more lethargic and do more sitting than walking. All of the lack of sleep side-effects will fundamentally have a negative effect on your ability to keep the weight off.

• • • • •

Sleeping is not overrated, and it is one of the basic facets of our life that we have to become aware of and more importantly, begin to manage if we want to live a balanced life. If we can make sleeping a priority instead of a privilege, we will become more balanced and perform at a much higher level in all the facets of our life!

It's perplexing for some of us to think that making more time for sleep will help with keeping the weight off, but hopefully now you can see how sleep affects our well-being in so many ways and has so much effect on our weight that it cannot be cut or under budget for very long before it shows up as a weight dilemma.

Our quantity and quality of sleep will determine how well we can balance our emotions and keep our energy levels high throughout the entire day so we can stay mentally focused on our weight-loss program. If your sleep facet isn't balanced and you're not able to get the recommended amount of sleep, then take a good look at how you can become more aware of your sleep patterns and better manage it. It's going to be a big factor in whether you're going to be successful with taking the weight off and keeping it off in the future.

S.M.A.R.T. SHIFT

Now it's time to create and implement your 7-Day *S.M.A.R.T. SHIFT* for the Sleep Facet! Please get a pen and take a couple of minutes to jot down which shift you could make to increase the quality and quantity of your sleep so you can rest, recover and keep the weight off!

Shift examples:

- Napping
- Reading before bed
- Turning off devices before bed
- Lights out rule!

What is your Simple/Stupid Shift?

How will you measure your success?

Is everything you will need accessible?

How will you reward yourself?

Who will you team up with to start this shift?

THE SIXTH FACET: SUBSTANCES

Josephine had been using prescribed anti-depressants to treat the depression she suffered from. Although the medication wasn't supposed to cause weight gain, she gained a considerable amount of weight after she started taking them.

After the first year of coaching, something remarkable happened. Josephine spoke to her doctor about a plan to reduce the anti-depressant medication and eventually discontinued taking it.

Reflecting on how this was possible, I could clearly see that the awareness, management and balance that Josephine was practicing in her F.E.A.R.S. not only allowed her to lose all of the weight and look like a completely different person physically, but it also changed her way of being. She was more upbeat, happy and energized. She didn't have any severe bouts of depression any longer, and she felt emotionally stable.

Since Josephine had balanced her 5-Facets and dealt with the underlying fear that her marriage break-up was causing her, she felt more confident and in control of her life because she had learned the practices to manage and balance her life. She is no longer needed a substance or a prescription drug to provide an artificial balance.

Substances could be considered legal or illegal, prescribed or self-prescribed. They could be used for alleviating a legitimate medical, physical or psychological condition and be considered medication. Many medications are used to correct imbalances in our bodies and brains such as our blood pressure, cholesterol, and mood. Other substances provide relief or an escape from emotional disturbances in our life or are used recreationally to enhance our mood in social settings.

Are you using any substances or medications and more importantly are they interfering with your overall balance? Are they causing any side-effects? Are they causing weight gain? Are they causing your F.E.A.R.S. to be symptomatic and out of balance? Could your medications be treating a problem that you could be possibly treating on your own by balancing your F.E.A.R.S. as we have been discussing?

If you have been prescribed medication for a medical condition and your doctor doesn't recommend ever discontinuing the treatment, then perhaps it wouldn't be wise to consider managing your medical condition without the medication. If you're using recreational substances in a responsible and balanced way, then you shouldn't have any concerns.

For the person that is using substances for relief or an escape from issues that they are dealing with (or not dealing with) in their lives, then I would ask you to consider investigating why you feel you need relief and an escape in the first place and what would it take to find a more natural form of relieving your stress.

In doing so, you can then have a whole new awareness of the real problem and begin to manage it by balancing your F.E.A.R.S. just as I did.

For the person like Josephine who was prescribed medications to balance her emotions, investigating why you're feeling depressed and working on correcting the imbalances in your 5-Facets, just as she did, may allow you with your doctor's approval to stop taking the medication.

MISTAKES PEOPLE MAKE
"Sometimes we are susceptible to
false expectations appearing real."

J osephine's weight-loss journey was a test because it meant for the first time she would have to consider herself as a priority if she expected to be successful this time with keeping the weight off. She would need to look into all 5-Facets of her lifestyle and do the work required to become aware, manage and balance all of them synergistically. This was Josephine's ultimate test in life thus far, and she passed with flying colors, but she did have a few falls and frustrations along the way.

Although Josephine lost 50 pounds in one year, it took another year for her body to adjust to her new weight so that her body could naturally regulate its metabolism to maintain her desired weight. Josephine had her share of slip-ups but none of which resulted in any serious damages or where she gained a substantial amount of the weight back. I realize now that if I had told her that she would need one year to lose the weight and one year for her new weight to stabilize, I'm not sure if she would have enrolled in my program.

Josephine told me that her expectation at the beginning of the program was to lose 50-60 pounds in three months. That would mean Josephine would need to lose 4-5 pounds per week. She had lost weight this rapidly with past diets so she assumed she would be able to do it again. Perhaps she could have repeated this kind of rapid weight-loss, but I knew that it wasn't sustainable.

On some weeks when she would see only one pound lost or less she would think that she was failing and become very frustrated. I would remind her of the journey she was on and of the vision she had for her new life which was not just about keeping the weight off but also about being able to look back in the mirror and be proud of the person she had become.

I also noticed a pattern in Josephine that whenever she didn't see the scale moving in a downward direction that matched her expectations, she would want to hit the panic button and go back to her old beliefs that she needed to be more strict, rigid and I might add, unrealistic with her diet and exercise. She would go back to her old way of thinking that less food and more activity in an exaggerated and unsustainable way would get her to the goal quicker. It was then that I would remind her that working harder wouldn't mean she would achieve her goal any faster, in fact, it would eventually sabotage our plan completely, and she would sooner or later gain the weight back.

I would also remind her that any shift or change we made within the 5-Facets of her lifestyle could be maintained forever. We used to have a saying that we would jokingly bring up whenever she would want to hit the panic button, which was "today and tomorrow." This meant that what she was doing today to lose the weight, she would need to do tomorrow, which implied forever, to keep the weight off. I reminded her that this is why it was so important to find practices that were a good fit for her to take the weight off and which could be sustained for the long-term.

As I mentioned she did have some digressions which occurred when she was trying to work something new into her life, like when she moved to a new home after her separation or when she took on a new career in the years that followed, or if she needed to work something out of her life like a relationship that wasn't serving her any longer and had become toxic and disruptive to her weight-loss program. These things would upset her schedule and all the systems she had in place to keep the weight off.

I would see these disruptions in her life by looking at her patterns. The first thing I would notice is that she would stop logging her food, then I would see her activity decrease and ultimately she would stop weighing herself. These were the early warning signs that there was a disruption going on in her life that she needed to deal with because it was showing up in her F.E.A.R.S.

In some of the most severe disturbances, such as when she separated from her husband, she would also become very isolated and would avoid communicating with me. She would be in a sense, hide-out and stay in the dark to avoid anything or anyone (including me) that would bring light to her crisis which would mean she would also need to commence dealing with it. Josephine would also feel the guilt and shame for not being able to deal with the issues in her life, which would cause her so much confusion and distraction that she just didn't have the capacity to focus on keeping the weight off.

The ironic thing is that when I finally contacted her, I was able to help balance her emotions and relieve her of much unnecessary self-imposed stress. I would coax her out of the dark and depressed state she had put herself in and bring in some well-needed light to let her see that the crisis she had been building by her reaction to the stress of the situation was not the big undefeatable mogul that she thought it was.

We began breaking it into its individual pieces and started working on reframing the situation into something smaller that she could work on one piece at a time. The priority was to turn her attention toward herself and fall back into the practices we had developed for her F.E.A.R.S., which gave her back a sense of control and allowed her to deal with life situations more effectively.

There is something so common that almost everyone of us who sets weight-loss expectations suffers from. It happens when setting weight-loss expectations that are unrealistic and unsustainable. This is when we face another type of F.E.A.R.S. (*False Expectations Appearing Real Syndrome*).

When you begin to believe in your false expectations, you unquestionably are going to feel stuck with your weight-loss and perhaps frustrated to the point that you feel like giving up entirely when these expectations aren't realized.

I don't want to see you ever get to that point so let's consider what false expectations are most common before you start your next - and last weight-loss program outlined in this book.

THE TOP 5 UNREALISTIC WEIGHT-LOSS EXPECTATIONS

1. EXPECTING IT TO BE FAST AND EASY

I know that you are in a hurry to accomplish your weight-loss goal. Why wouldn't you be, you've suffered for long enough, and now you have made a decision to change, make corrections and take the weight off.

I support you 100% with this decision, but the deadlines you may have given yourself could be unrealistic. Losing 1-2 pounds of weight per week is the standard average that almost all weight-loss professionals including those in the medical field agree with. Although you might not want to believe this truth and perhaps you have even proved it to be false in the past, I would ask you to consider if you kept the weight off when you lost it rapidly? There is no cheating this biological law without invasive medical intervention.

After reading this book, hopefully, you will know that we can't beat our body's biology. Eventually, it will always win, and you will gain all the weight back. It's inevitable because we're fighting against our nature.

It will also take you a considerable period to re-balance your body and mind so that you will be less susceptible to putting the weight back on. There are biological and behavioral balances that will take the time to realign. Through my personal and hundreds of client experiences, the typical timeframe for these adjustments to occur is one year. It is after one year of you keeping the weight off successfully that your chances of keeping it off for good will be permanent or as long as you keep your F.E.A.R.S. in balance.

If this seems too long of a period for you to accept, another perspective would be to ask yourself how long did it take to put on the weight in the first place? If I can speak candidly with you, how long have you neglected yourself which itself has created a weight problem? Now in all reasonableness, how long will it take to make all the necessary changes, solve your weight problem and keep the weight off forever? Would you expect this to be a process that will require you to show yourself some patience?

On a personal note, it took me one year to take off 50 pounds and one year for my new weight to stabilize. I have kept the weight off ever since.

Just The Facts:

The NWCR study states "Individuals who had kept their weight off for two years or more had markedly increased odds of continuing to maintain their weight over the following year. This finding is encouraging because it suggests that, if individuals can succeed at maintaining their weight loss for two years, they can reduce their risk of subsequent regain by nearly 50%." (Wing, R. Rena and Suzanne Phelan, Long-term weight loss maintenance 1'2'3'4, *The American Journal of Clinical Nutrition,* vol. 82, no. 1, pp. 224S).

2. EXPECTING THAT DIET AND EXERCISE WILL KEEP THE WEIGHT OFF

Most of our belief system on how to successfully keep the weight off will have us looking for the solution in diet and exercise alone. This is mainly because of the propaganda that the weight-loss industry has ingrained in us.

The truth is that to keep the weight off you will need to be aware, manage and balance not just two facets, but all of your 5-Facets.

As my friend Dr. Isaac Jones from Designer Health Centers stated, many of us have developed a lot of "B.S" or Bad-Belief Systems which we will now need to eradicate so we can adopt a belief system that matches reality and serves our new desires of not just losing the weight—but keeping it off forever.

3. EXPECTING TO HAVE NO SLIPS OR SETBACKS

I have realized in our society that we can be our worst critics, and sometimes we can turn into our worst enemy. We seem to have expectations of ourselves that require us to be pretty much perfect with everything we do, and when we don't live up to that expectation, or we have a slip and a setback, many times we beat ourselves up to a level that nobody else could unleash on us.

Through my eye-witness accounts, it's the slips and falls that people encounter while on a weight-loss program that creates a slippery downward spiral that leads to a place in someone's life that they feel it is impossible to recover from.

Given that many people expect weight-loss to be a quick and easy process, they firmly believe they won't encounter any setbacks. The reality is that you are not perfect, nobody is. You are going to slip and fall, but if you can pick yourself up as soon as you do, you will recover from any obstacle you may face. The trick is not to hide from it or be afraid of it. Remember that this is supposed to happen. You're supposed to have setbacks, so you have an opportunity to reset and do it correctly the next time or the next time after that (if you're a proud graduate from the school of hard knocks like me). After I finished rehab they told me that I would have relapses and that this was to be expected—well I'm telling you the same thing now. You are going to have relapses in your weight-loss program that will appear initially as a setback but if you don't give up what you will later see is that this temporary defeat was a necessary step to see what you can do differently and more effectively.

Just The Facts:

The NWCR study also states that "Preventing small regains from turning into larger relapses appears critical to recovery among successful weight losers." (Wing, R. Rena and Suzanne Phelan, Long-term weight loss maintenance 1'2'3'4, *The American Journal of Clinical Nutrition*, vol. 82, no. 1, pp. 225S).

4. EXPECTING TO DO IT ALONE

The problem with expecting to do it on your own is the lack of accountability. By nature, we're prone to being more accountable to others than to ourselves. Knowing the challenges you will face with weight-loss, having only to be accountable to yourself and nobody else (although this might feel more comfortable to you) will result in a higher failure rate. If you were accountable to yourself then how did you develop a weight problem in the first place?

The resistance that I see in most is their inability to accept help from others. It seems to be a cultural phenomenon because we certainly don't appear to have been created to be independent DIYers. We are taught at a young age to be independent and that we can do it on our own, but this is in conflict with our true human nature. We are a social species, and we need social support to get through challenges and to make the necessary positive changes in our life. Nobody that I know has ever done anything worth mentioning completely on their own.

I also was very resistant to accept assistance in the past. In fact, I attribute this to be a character flaw that prolonged my past struggle. It was when I raised my hand and said "Hey I need some help here, I don't know how to get myself out of this mess, would you mind helping me out, I'd appreciate it" that my life took a sharp turn in an upward trajectory.

Support comes in many forms and is available to you, so you don't have to go it alone. Family, friends, co-workers can all be recruited for support if you can conjure up the courage to tell them that you want to lose the weight and keep it off this time. Most people are pleasantly surprised by the positive reaction we get when we can show some honesty and humility with the people in our circle.

I would also recommend that you consider investigating and investing in a guide for this important life endeavor. This will save you time, money and effort, but be cautious on whom you choose because this will be the person in whom you will invest all of your trust to create a clear path toward your goal.

Guides are people such as coaches, doctors, and nutritionists. These people not only provide the professional support that many of us can benefit from but also provide you with the structure or the program. They also administer the highest level of accountability and give you the timelines and deadlines to keep you in successful momentum.

Even though I am a coach, I have a coach because I too need support and structure for all of the aspirations I want to fulfill in my life. He leads me in the right direction as it is difficult to steer and navigate at the same time.

I also wanted to let you know that the only reason you're reading this book right now is that of my writing coach Angela Lauria and her program, the Author Incubator, which enabled me to fulfill my dream of writing a book.

Just The Facts:

The NWCR study mentions "Interestingly, about one-half (55.4%) reported receiving some help with weight loss (commercial program, physician, nutritionist), whereas the others (44.6%) reported losing the weight entirely on their own." (Wing, R. Rena and Suzanne Phelan, Long-term weight loss maintenance 1'2'3'4, *The American Journal of Clinical Nutrition,* vol. 82, no. 1, pp. 223S).

5. EXPECTING HOW YOU TOOK IT OFF –WON'T BE HOW YOU'LL KEEP IT OFF

I have watched people make this mistake time and time again, and it hurts every time I see it. Many people have set their weight-loss program completely around their weight-loss goal. Because of this, they believe that they must push harder and faster so the only solutions are radical changes they can make with their diet and exercise that will not be sustainable.

Their approach would work if it were true that once your weight-loss goal is achieved you can put your feet up and never have to worry about your weight ever again. Knowing with certainty that we will be obligated and responsible for maintaining our weight in the future, there is only one possible solution to ensure that the lifestyle we create to lose the weight is sustainable to keep the weight off in the future: as Stephen Covey said in habit two from his famous book *The Seven Habits of Highly Successful People*, we need to "Begin with the End in Mind."

Whenever I've learned that someone has lost weight and has been able to maintain it for a year or more, I become very intrigued and always ask them how they did it and what they're doing to keep it off. They never tell me about some cutting-edge scientific diet that they started or some insane exercise regime; rather they reveal the simple shifts they made within their lifestyle that enabled them to lose it and keep it off. This is a testament to what I have known for years: How you take it off will be how you keep it off.

Just The Facts:

In summary, findings from the NWCR registry suggest "six key strategies for long-term success at weight loss" which include:

1. Engaging in high levels of physical activity
2. Eating a diet that is low in calories and fat
3. Eating breakfast
4. Self-monitoring weight on a regular basis
5. Maintaining a consistent eating pattern throughout the week and on weekends
6. Catching "slips" before they turn into larger regains

(Wing, R. Rena and Suzanne Phelan, Long-term weight loss maintenance 1'2'3'4, *The American Journal of Clinical Nutrition*, vol. 82, no. 1, pp. 225S).

MY WISH FOR YOU

"If you want to become a butterfly you
must be willing to break through your
shell, spread your wings and learn to fly."

I was overwhelmed with emotion when Josephine surprised me one day at the office. She stood before me, not as the same woman I had met three years earlier.

Josephine now had an aura that surrounded her and beamed brightly everywhere she went. She had a type of genuine confidence that you only achieve when you've invested in yourself and truly know what your self-worth is. From the way she dressed, talked and walked. Everything seemed to be an authentic expression of who she truly was. She was finally able to look herself in the mirror and feel a sense of pride in her reflection.

Josephine was no longer hiding in the shadows of despair. Instead, she was radiating light into everyone's life. She was now living the life she had always dreamed of. As she took care of herself, everything else seemed to take care of itself.

Josephine hadn't changed who she was; she just discovered who she truly was. She was always in there but hidden under layers of weight and underlying fears. She used to say she felt like something was missing in her life, and now I knew what that was—it was the real Josephine.

After she had left, I returned to my desk and found a card that Josephine had written

Kris,
Thank you for being such a great coach and mentor. I've learned so much from this program I don't know where to begin. It's taught me self worth which I struggled with for so many years as well as self forgiveness. You've taught me the skills and showed me the tools that I'll have always with me to handle all of lifes challenging moments and achieve all of my goals. Thank You
Thank you again
Josephine

Now it's your turn to become aware of your F.E.A.R.S. so you can begin to manage and balance your life.

Now is your time to keep the weight off, so you are no longer weighed down.

This is your time to shine. You have no idea how proud I am of you for taking this courageous step to keep the weight off forever.

Keep your head out of the sand and in the clouds. Dream. Believe and Inspire to Aspire.

With love,

Kris J. Simpson

ACKNOWLEDGEMENTS

Writing a book has been a decade-long dream for me. This dream included many doubts and fears that had always stopped me in the past from even getting started. The experience of publishing my first book has been a birthing process where I have felt pain, elation and even shed a few tears of gratitude along the way. As this book grew, it took on an identity of its own. I now wish to express my gratitude for those that inspired the All-Inclusive Diet into creation.

I know that this book would never have been born if I didn't get straight and sober. My father was one of my biggest supporters through this process. He was the strong shoulder that I leaned on while I was still on shaky ground. He now tells me how proud he is of me every chance he gets.

My mother the retired librarian and children's book writer who instilled in me her love for books and writing. Although I took my path through Stephen King's *Pet Cemetery*, it was her that first introduced me to one of my first and favorite books *Oh, The Places You'll Go* by Dr. Seuss. Ironically this was also the book that they read to us on the day I left rehab. Through my eternal connection to my mother, I feel as though she has co-authored this book.

Tony Sansotta or "Uncle T." has been my mentor since I was in grade school. He has been by my side through every life challenge I have experienced and every success I have ever achieved. The greatest thing he ever taught me was to take care of the important things, myself and my family, and everything else would take care of itself. He was right.

It was Amanda and her ability to step into the shoes of my ideal reader who became my loyal and loving confidant while I wrote this book. Our breakfast brainstorm sessions fueled by egg-white omelets, vegetables, fruit, a single serving of coffee for her and multiple servings for me hashed out the content of this book and gave me memories I will cherish forever.

My long time friend Giovanni Marsico, the founder of the Archangel Academy was the first person I told about my decade-long dream to write a book. He was committed to helping me and along with all of the great resources and advice he offered me, Giovanni also said that he believed in me. That was worth its weight in gold. I will always remember our trip to the bookstore and standing in front of the health and fitness section where he declared: "And the name of your book shall be the All-Inclusive Diet." And so it was.

I asked my friend and courage coach Billy Anderson what I should write my book about, and he answered my question with a question: "What was the most challenging struggle you were able to overcome in your life? Well, that's what you should be writing about". I found the courage and followed his advice.

Thank you to Caroline Krikorian, Dan Falconio, Nat Augursa and the big crew at Bodies By Design who took care of business so I could pursue my passion and author my first book.

A big hug for my publisher Angela Lauria who introduced me to my inner author through her book-writing program the Author Incubator. Special thanks to my editor Cynthia Kane.

Lastly and most importantly, thank-you to the *Freedom 13* clients that I have had the privilege of not only teaching and coaching, but who have also let me be a student and taught me everything I needed to know about keeping the weight off. Special mention to Freedom Fighters, Anna Lopes, Susan Kwolek, Nadia Butera, Tatiana Jaku, Catti Rodriguez, Rose Tersigni and Mary Mete.

With Gratitude,

Kris J. Simpson

ABOUT THE AUTHOR

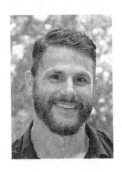 Kris J. Simpson is a veteran of the weight-loss, fitness, and physical rehabilitation industry. As an elite personal trainer, former national bodybuilding champion and present CEO and founder of *Bodies By Design Fitness Studios*, Kris is recognized as a weight-loss and fitness guru and his expertise and wisdom is in high demand. He was also featured as a spokesperson for health and fitness on CP24, City TV, and the E! Channel.

As a Weight-loss Coach, Seminar Leader, Speaker, and Author, Kris found his calling to help other people restore balance and keep the weight off as he did for himself. Kris spreads the weight-loss and wellness gospel by dedicating his life to this cause. As he sets his sights on the future, his crusade will continue by showing others how to keep the weight off and sharing his vision of the health and fitness experience with his clients and the world at large. As his motto states, he will continue to—*Inspire to Aspire*™

Happy Words From *Freedom 13* Clients

"I'm down 80 pounds and if I were to describe everything I took away from this program I would be writing a novel. All I can say is thank you, Kris! You've opened my eyes, given me an opportunity to rediscover myself and to be happy, fearless and free!!"

—Tatiana J.

"I am now physically, mentally, and emotionally stronger. By taking care of myself, I found freedom, inner peace, calmness, and contentment. This, in turn, has helped me to take better care of my family, which is what I was always aiming to do. I'm still doing what I was doing before and probably more, but feeling less stressed. Kris helped me to realize that it's okay to have 'me' time and that I needed to take care of myself too!"

— Nadia B.

"Kris and the *Freedom 13* program taught me how to look within myself to find inner peace and calm. I went looking for one thing but found something better. After many hours of self-reflection, it's helped and continues to help me to be more aware of my emotions and how to better respond rather than react when life presents me with challenging situations. Thankfully I feel I have the tools now to help me stay on track and keep the weight off!"

— Rose T.

Thank You

This isn't the end, but rather the beginning of your weight-loss & wellness journey and I would love to guide you every step of the way!

Please download all of the tools that you will need for your journey at www.krisjsimpson.com/free-downloads

I can always be reached through my website at www.krisjsimpson.com or at kris@krisjsimpson.com so please get in touch with your questions and comments.

If you're ready to take the next step and work with me, please visit www.krisjsimpson.com for more information about my programs and how to get started!

A free eBook edition is available with the purchase of this book.

To claim your free eBook edition:

1. Download the Shelfie app.
2. Write your name in upper case in the box.
3. Use the Shelfie app to submit a photo.
4. Download your eBook to any device.

Shelfie

A free eBook edition is available
with the purchase of this print book.

CLEARLY PRINT YOUR NAME ABOVE IN UPPER CASE

Instructions to claim your free eBook edition:
1. Download the Shelfie app for Android or iOS
2. Write your name in **UPPER CASE** above
3. Use the Shelfie app to submit a photo
4. Download your eBook to any device

Print & Digital Together Forever.

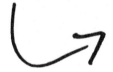

Snap a photo   Free eBook   Read anywhere

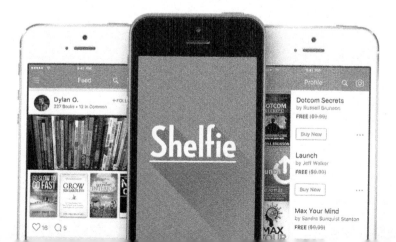

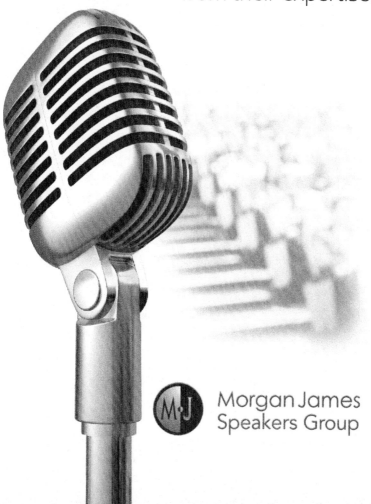

www.TheMorganJamesSpeakersGroup.com

We connect Morgan James published authors with live and online events and audiences whom will benefit from their expertise.

Morgan James
Speakers Group

Morgan James makes all of our titles available
through the Library for All Charity Organizations.

www.LibraryForAll.org

CPSIA information can be obtained
at www.ICGtesting.com
Printed in the USA
LVOW03s0106040517
533192LV00001B/157/P